OXFORD SPECIALTY TRAINING

How to pass the MRCS OSCE

Volume 2

OXFORD SPECIALTY TRAINING

How to pass the MRCS OSCE
Volume 2

EDITED BY

Jowan Penn-Barwell

Charlie Docker

OXFORD
UNIVERSITY PRESS

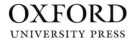

OXFORD
UNIVERSITY PRESS

Great Clarendon Street, Oxford OX2 6DP

Oxford University Press is a department of the University of Oxford.
It furthers the University's objective of excellence in research, scholarship,
and education by publishing worldwide in

Oxford New York

Auckland Cape Town Dar es Salaam Hong Kong Karachi
Kuala Lumpur Madrid Melbourne Mexico City Nairobi
New Delhi Shanghai Taipei Toronto

With offices in

Argentina Austria Brazil Chile Czech Republic France Greece
Guatemala Hungary Italy Japan Poland Portugal Singapore
South Korea Switzerland Thailand Turkey Ukraine Vietnam

Oxford is a registered trade mark of Oxford University Press
in the UK and in certain other countries

Published in the United States
by Oxford University Press Inc., New York

© Oxford University Press 2011

British Library Cataloguing in Publication Data
Data available

Library of Congress Cataloging in Publication Data
Data available

Typeset by Glyph International, Bangalore, India
Printed in Great Britain
on acid-free paper by
Ashford Colour Press Ltd, Gosport, Hampshire

ISBN 978-0-19-958300-3

10 9 8 7 6 5 4 3 2 1

For Julie, Lotte, and JJ (CD)
For Bill and Janie (JPB)

Foreword

The Objective Structured Clinical Examination is now in its third year as part of the MRCS examination. The name means what it says. There should be no unfair variation in questioning and the topics tested in each session must be the same for all candidates. This does not mean that the standard of the examination is any different from the previous free questioning nor is the syllabus narrower.

While focussed on the type of testing found in the OSCE stations, this book is in fact a comprehensive textbook, incorporating basic science and clinical surgery, not in a didactic way, but presenting real life practical scenarios. The authors present their experience in a highly practical way. Do not be put off by the apparent stress on 'communication skills'. This may be the spirit of the age but this book also gives young doctors and even medical students plenty of relevant facts to communicate!

Candidates for the MRCS and others studying this book will not only learn enough to pass the examination but will also be equipped with the basic knowledge to start their careers as specialist trainees.

John Black
March 2010

Contents

Contents

List of contributors

Editors

Jowan G. Penn-Barwell MRCS
Trauma and Orthopaedic Registrar, Royal Navy

Charlie Docker FRCS (T&O)
Consultant Trauma and Orthopaedic Surgeon, Worcestershire Acute Hospitals NHS Trust

Authors

Part 1: Trunk and Thorax

Robert W. Jordan MRCS
ST1 Trauma and Orthopaedics, West Midlands Deanery

Joseph Papanikitas MRCS
ST2 General Surgery, West Midlands Deanery

Andy Robinson MB ChB
ST2 General Surgery, West Midlands Deanery

Part 2: Limbs and Spine

Jowan G. Penn-Barwell MRCS
Trauma and Orthopaedic Registrar, Royal Navy

Part 3: Head and Neck

Caroline Mary Mann MRCS
Registrar Emergency Medicine, Hawke's Bay Hospital, Hawkes Bay District Health Board, New Zealand

Part 4: Neuroscience

Desiré G. Ngoga MRCS
ST4 Neurosurgery, West Midlands Deanery

Stuart Roberts MRCS
ST3 Neurosurgery, West Midlands Deanery
with contributions by **Robert W. Jordan** MRCS *and* **Caroline Mary Mann** MRCS

Original illustrations

Kannan T. Periyasamy MD MSc Surg. Diploma IC

Acronyms and abbreviations

AAA	abdominal aortic aneurysm
ACE	angiotensin converting enzyme
ADH	antidiuretic hormone (vasopressin)
AFP	alpha-fetoprotein
AP	anteroposterior
APB	abductor pollicis brevis
APL	abductor pollicis longus
ARDS	acute respiratory distress syndrome
ASIS	anterior superior iliac spine
ATLS	Advanced Trauma Life Support™
AV	atrioventricular
AVM	arteriovenous malformations
AXR	abdominal radiograph
BCC	basal cell carcinoma
ßHCG	beta-human chorionic gonadotropin
BMR	basal metabolic rate
BOO	bladder outlet obstruction
BPH	benign prostatic hypertrophy
CCA	common carotid artery
CEA	carcinoembryonic antigen
CIS	carcinoma *in situ*
CMCJ	carpometacarpal joint
CNS	central nervous system
CO	cardiac output
CPP	cerebral perfusion pressure
CRP	C-reactive protein
CSF	cerebrospinal fluid
CXR	chest radiograph
DIPJ	distal interphalangeal joint
DRE	digital rectal examination
DSA	digital subtraction angiogram
EBV	Epstein–Barr virus
ECA	external carotid artery
ECG	electrocardiogram
ECRB	extensor carpi radialis brevis
ECRL	extensor carpi radialis longus
ECU	extensor carpi ulnaris
EDC	extensor digitorum communis
EDM	extensor digiti minimi
EEG	electroencephalogram
EHL	extensor hallucis longus
EJV	external jugular vein
ENT	ear, nose and throat
EPB	extensor pollicis brevis

EPL	extensor pollicis longus
ERCP	endoscopic retrograde cholangiopancreatography
ESR	erythrocyte sedimentation rate
EUS	endoscopic ultrasound
EVD	external ventricular drainage
FAP	familial adenomatous polyposis
FBC	full blood count
FCR	flexor carpi radialis
FCU	flexor carpi ulnaris
FDP	flexor digitorum profundus
FDS	flexor digitorum superficialis
FFA	free fatty acids
FNA(C)	fine needle aspiration (and cytology)
FPB	flexor pollicis brevis
FPL	flexor pollicis longus
GA	general anaesthetic
GCS	Glasgow Coma Scale
GIT	gastrointestinal tract
GORD	gastro-oesophageal reflux disease
GTN	glyceryl trinitrate
HCG	human chorionic gonadotropin
HIV	human immunodeficiency virus
ICA	internal carotid artery
ICP	intracranial pressure
IJV	internal jugular vein
IMA	inferior mesenteric artery
INR	international normalized ratio
IPJ	interphalangeal joint
IV	intravenous
IVC	inferior vena cava
IVH	intraventricular haemorrhage
JVP	jugular venous pressure
KUB	kidney, ureters, bladder (radiograph)
LA	local anaesthetic
LBO	large-bowel obstruction
LCCA	Left common carotid artery
LDH	lactate dehydrogenase
LFT	liver function test
LH	luteinizing hormone
LHRH	luteinizing hormone releasing hormone
LIF	left iliac fossa
LP	lumbar puncture
LP	lumbo-peritoneal
LUTS	lower urinary tract symptoms

MCA	middle cerebral artery
MCPJ	metacarpophalangeal joint
MEN	multiple endocrine neoplasia
MI	myocardial infarction
MNG	multinodular goitre
MRC	Medical Research Council
MRCP	magnetic resonance cholangiopancreatography
MRI	magnetic resonance imaging
MS	multiple sclerosis
MSU	mid-stream urinalysis
MTPJ	metatarsophalangeal joint
MVAC	methotrexate, vinblastine, adriamycin, cisplatin
NBM	nil by mouth
NG	nasogastric
NHL	non-Hodgkin's lymphoma
NSAIDs	non-steroidal anti-inflammatory drugs
NSGCT	nonseminoma germ cell tumor
OA	osteoarthritis
OD	once daily
ORIF	open reduction, internal fixation
PAN	polyarteritis nodosa
PET	positron emission tomography
PID	pelvic inflammatory disease
PIPJ	proximal interphalangeal joint
PP	pancreatic polypeptide
PQ	pronator quadratus
PR	per rectum
PSA	prostate specific antigen
PT	pronator teres
PT	prothrombin time
PTC	percutaneous transhepatic cholangiogram
PTH	parathyroid hormone
RA	right atrium
RBC	red blood cell
RhA	rheumatoid arthritis
RIF	right inguinal fossa
RLN	recurrent laryngeal nerve
RoM	range of movement
RUQ	right upper quadrant
SA	sinoatrial
SAH	subarachnoid haemorrhage
SBO	small-bowel obstruction
SCC	squamous cell carcinoma
SCLC	small-cell lung cancer
SCM	sternocleidomastoid muscle
SERM	selective oestrogen receptor modulator.
SIADH	syndrome of inappropriate antidiuretic hormone hypersecretion

SLE	systemic lupus erythematosus
SMA	superior mesenteric artery
SVC	superior vena cava
TB	tuberculosis
TCC	transitional cell carcinoma
TFT	thyroid function test
THRH	thyroid hormone releasing hormone
TIA	transient ischaemic attack
TMJ	temporomandibular joint
TNM	tumour, node and metastasis
TOE	trans-oesophageal echocardiogram
TPN	total parenteral nutrition
TSH	thyroid stimulating hormone
TTE	transthoracic echocardiogram
TUR	transurethral resection
TURBT	transurethral resection of bladder tumour
TURP	trans-urethral resection of prostate
TWOC	trial without catheter
U&Es	urea and electrolytes
USS	ultrasound scan
UTI	urinary tract infection
UV	ultraviolet
VA	ventriculo-atrial
VATS	video assisted thoracoscopic surgery
VP	ventriculo-peritoneal
WFNS	World Federation of Neurological Surgeons
WHO	World Health Organization

Introduction

Welcome to the second volume of *How to pass the MRCS OSCE*. This book is designed and written especially for the new intercollegiate MRCS Part B Objective Structured Clinical Exam (OSCE). Our intention is that this book should help candidates convert the knowledge they will have already acquired in hospital and from textbooks into the form that the examiners will be trying to elicit. This book will not replace the time you need to spend with the anatomy atlas and the skeleton, or attending extra clinics or watching prosection DVDs. It will, however, be a very time-efficient way to refine the knowledge that those activities provide in the final weeks leading up to your MRCS Part B.

This volume is focused on the 50% of the examination stations that are themed to specific areas. MRCS Part B is the first time that the MRCS examination process has allowed candidates to chose two areas to 'major' and 'minor' in. It is important that candidates realize that they will be examined on areas across the entire syllabus and that they will not be asked questions in the chosen areas in any greater depth, just that they will spend a greater proportion of the examination being questioned on these areas. It is also important that in their preparation candidates do not equate a speciality area to a surgical speciality; 'Limbs and Spine', is not orthopaedics—you may well be asked about Hunter's canal and vascular problems in a 'Limbs and Spine' station. The MRCS examines breadth rather than depth and, as the OSCE title states, it has to be objective with every candidate having as similar an experience as possible. Exceptional performances in one station no longer make up for poor performances in others.

Formally, the MRCS syllabus combines the syllabuses of the constituent Royal Colleges. However, there has been a significant shift in the emphasis of the material that comes up in the MRCS Part B when compared to older formats. Pure physiology now receives less focus, apart from the applied physiology of critical care, and non-neuroscience embryology has largely disappeared. In recognition that candidates' surgical experience is much narrower with the demise of Basic Surgical Training rotations, candidates are no longer expected to describe how to perform a range of operations; they are, however, expected to be confident in describing certain life-saving procedures such as chest drain insertion or venous cutdown. Knowledge and skills from essential training, such as the Foundation Programme (in the UK) and Basic Surgical Skill Course can be considered potential examination material.

This book contains only a few good-quality pictures; this is because this volume is not intended to teach you the material, but help you to structure your answers in a form that makes it easier for the examiners to award you marks. Since the stations require verbal or occasionally written answers we felt that presenting information visually would not help candidates recall and relay this back to the examiners. As mentioned earlier, you will be reading this book with considerable knowledge and experience already, probably more than you think. You will learn better if you relate the material in the book back to this knowledge and experience. We have highlighted key knowledge in the coloured boxes: **grey** for *aide memoires* and **purple** for points that are particularly relevant to the examination. Add your own notes and pictures. Make this book your own to fall back on in the last few days before the exam.

Finally, good luck! This examination is hard. If it was not, you would not feel the pride that hopefully you will do the day you first introduce yourself as Mr or Miss or write MRCS after your name. Most new college members remark on the difference in the way they are treated as a surgical trainee after they have passed, with a greater sense of inclusion by their seniors which often translates into being allowed to do far more in theatre. This is partly due to your having proved your commitment to the profession of surgery and partly to the fact that in acquiring the knowledge required to pass MRCS you will be a better doctor and more competent surgical trainee. Once again, good luck!

Jowan Penn-Barwell MRCS
Charlie Docker FRCS(T&O)

PART 1
TRUNK AND THORAX

Section 1 **Anatomy**

Chapter 1 **Torso surface anatomy**

This topic is easily introduced in the MRCS examination, and in a variety of ways. A candidate's knowledge of surface anatomy and vertebral levels can be assessed with reference to a live model, a prosected specimen, or CT/MR images.

1.1 Thoracic surface anatomy

Anatomical lines

Midclavicular line	Vertical line down from middle of clavicle
Anterior axillary line	Vertical line along the anterior axillary fold (formed by pectoralis major)
Midaxillary line	Runs parallel to the anterior axillary line from apex of the axilla
Posterior axillary line	Vertical line along the posterior axillary fold (formed by latissimus dorsi and teres major)

Boundaries of the thoracic cage

Posterior	Thoracic vertebra
Lateral	Ribs and intercostal spaces
Anterior	Sternum and costal cartilages
Superior	Thoracic inlet—1st thoracic vertebra, 1st rib, and manubrium sternum
Inferior	Thoracic outlet—12th vertebra, xiphisternum, 12th rib, and diaphragm

Trachea

Commences at lower border of cricoid cartilage (C6) as a continuation of the larynx, enters thorax through the thoracic inlet before dividing at the angle of Louis (T4/5) into the two main bronchi.

Surface markings of pleura and lungs

> This area is often introduced in questions after a candidate has been asked to comment on a chest radiograph.

Pleura

* Apex of pleura projects 2.5 cm above the medial third of the clavicle.
* Line of pleural reflection passes behind the sternoclavicular joints and meet in the midline at the sternal angle.
* Right pleura passes inferiorly to the 6th costal cartilage.
* Left pleura passes laterally at the 4th costal cartilage and descends vertically lateral to the sternal border to the 6th costal cartilage.
* From the two points above, both pleura pass posteriorly crossing the 8th rib in the midclavicular line, the 10th in the midaxillary line reaching the level of the 12th posteriorly.

Lungs

Oblique fissure	Line drawn from a point 2.5 cm lateral to the 5th thoracic spinous process to the 6th costal cartilage anteriorly
Transverse fissure	Line drawn horizontally from the fourth costal cartilage to a point where it intersects the oblique fissure of the right lung

Heart

Left border	2nd left costal cartilage at sternal edge to 5th costal cartilage at midclavicular line (apex); formed mainly by left ventricle
Inferior border	6th right costal cartilage at sternal edge to the apex; formed by right ventricle and apical part of left ventricle
Right border	3rd right costal cartilage to 6th costal cartilage both at sternal edge; formed by right atrium

Valves

All the valves lie behind the sternum.

Aortic   Left border of sternum at level of 3rd intercostal space

Pulmonary   Left border of sternum at level of 3rd costal cartilage

Tricuspid   Behind midline of sternum at level of 4th costal cartilage

Mitral   Left border of sternum at 4th costal cartilage

It is important to remember that the site of valves differs from the optimum area for auscultation:

↗ **Aortic**   2nd costal cartilage at right sternal border

↗ **Pulmonary** 2nd costal cartilage at left sternal border

↗ **Tricuspid** 5th intercostal space left sternal border

↗ **Mitral**   5th intercostal space at left midclavicular line

---

1.2 Thoracic vertebral levels

The ribs should be identified from the 2nd costal cartilage which articulates with the sternum at the angle of Louis. Although the spinous processes of all thoracic vertebra can be palpated in the midline, the first palpable is the C7.

Vertebral levels of surface markings

T2   Superior angle of the scapula

T2/3   • Suprasternal notch
           • Spine of the scapula

T4/5   Sternal angle

T8   Inferior angle of scapula

T9   Xiphisternal joint

L3   Subcostal plane

Level of diaphragm openings and contents

T8   Inferior vena cava and right phrenic nerve

T10   Oesophagus, branches of the left gastric artery and vein, right phrenic nerve

T12   Aorta, thoracic duct, and azygos vein

At the level of the sternal angle there is an important 'transverse thoracic plane'; it acts as the division between the superior and inferior mediastinum. You should be able to discuss important thoracic features at this level:

↗ Beginning and end of the aortic arch

↗ Formation of the superior vena cava

↗ Bifurcation of the trachea

↗ Bifurcation of the pulmonary trunk

↗ Drainage of thoracic duct into the left brachiocephalic vein

---

1.3 Abdominal surface markings

On the surface, the abdomen has superior and inferior boundaries; however, be aware that the abdominal cavity extends superiorly under the ribs and inferiorly into the pelvis, offering some protection to the abdominal viscera.

Superior Costal margin which runs from 7th costal cartilage at xiphoid to tip of 12th rib

Inferior Inguinal ligament runs between anterior superior iliac spine to the pubic tubercle

You need to be familiar with the commonly used terms that divide the abdomen into quadrants or nine divisions:

Quadrants
- Horizontal line through umbilicus
- Vertical line through midline

Divisions
- Two midclavicular lines
- Two horizontal planes—subcostal and transtubercular

1.4 Visceral surface anatomy

Liver
- Lies in right upper quadrant and may just be palpable in normal individual on deep inspiration
- Lower border: tip of right 10th rib to left intercostal space in midclavicular line
- Upper border: horizontal line at the level of the 5th intercostal space

Kidney
- Hilum lies near transpyloric plane
- Upper pole is situated under the 11th and 12th ribs
- Lower pole can sometimes be palpated
- The right kidney lies around 2.5 cm (1 inch) lower than the left

Spleen
- Lies superficially in left hypochondrium between 9th and 11th ribs

Pancreas
- Not palpable
- Neck of pancreas overlies the 1st and 2nd lumbar vertebra at transpyloric plane
- Head lies to the right and inferiorly, the tail to the left and superiorly

1.5 Abdominal vertebral levels

When describing levels in the abdomen you can use easily identifiable structures to help orient yourself: the xiphisternum (T9) and the umbilicus (L3/4). There are three common planes that you should be aware of and be confident discussing—transpyloric, subcostal, and supracristal.

Transpyloric plane (L1)
- Halfway between suprasternal notch and pubis
- Passes through pylorus, duodenojejunal flexure, fundus of gallbladder, hila of kidneys, neck of pancreas, origin of superior mesenteric artery, and termination of the spinal cord

Transpyloric plane is a very common examination topic, often introduced with a CT image at the level of L1.

Subcostal plane (L3)

- ↗ Horizontal line joining lowest parts of thoracic cage
- ↗ Passes through the origin of inferior mesenteric artery

Supracristal plane (L4)

- ↗ Identified by horizontal line connecting most superior aspect of iliac crests, suprasternal notch and pubis
- ↗ Level of bifurcation of aorta and useful landmark when performing lumbar puncture

Vascular vertebral levels

The aorta enters the abdominal cavity through the diaphragm at the level of T12, it descends on the posterior abdominal wall before bifurcation at L4. Branches and their vertebral levels are commonly asked in the exam:

Coeliac axis	T12
Superior mesenteric artery	L1
Inferior mesenteric artery	L3

Chapter 2 **Chest and abdominal wall**

This topic commonly crops up in the MRCS examination as questions can easily be linked to practical stations, specimens, skeletons, and scans. Knowledge of the anatomy remains crucial in surgical practice when positioning and performing incisions.

2.1 Chest wall

The thoracic wall is mainly made up of skeletal and muscular components. Its cavity encloses the two pleura and the mediastinum and communicates with the neck and abdomen through apertures:

Components of thoracic wall

Posterior   12 thoracic vertebra + discs

Anterior   Sternum + costal cartilages

Laterally   Ribs + three intercostal muscles

Apertures

Superior boundaries   T1 vertebra, 1st rib+ manubrium

Inferior boundaries   T12 vertebra, 12th rib, xiphoid

Closed by diaphragm

Sternum

Consists of three major elements:

Manubrium
- Has suprasternal notch superiorly
- Articulates with the clavicle, 1st rib and upper half of 2nd rib

Body   Articulates with lower half of 2nd rib, 3rd to 6th ribs and upper half of 7th rib

Xiphoid process   Articulates with lower half of 7th rib

Anterior articulation:
- ⤢ 'True ribs' (I–VII) with sternum
- ⤢ 'False ribs' (VII–IX) to superior costal cartilages
- ⤢ 'Floating ribs' (XI+XII) no anterior articulation

Ribs

- ⤢ Provide attachments for muscles of neck, abdomen, back, and upper limbs
- ⤢ Typical rib has a head (with two facets), neck, tubercle (with facet), angle, and shaft with subcostal groove

Costovertebral joint   Two facets on head articulate with corresponding vertebra and one above

Costotransverse joint   Two synovial joint between rib tubercle and vertebral transverse process

1st rib

- ⤢ Unique, and a favourite exam question
- ⤢ Short, flat and increased curvature
- ⤢ Has a single facet for articulation with T1 vertebra
- ⤢ Has prominent tubercle where scalenus anterior inserts and this helps define course of important vessels:
  - Subclavian vein runs anterior to tubercle
  - Subclavian artery and lowest trunk of brachial plexus run posterior to tubercle

What is the sequence of layers when inserting a chest drain?

⤢ Skin

⤢ Superficial fascia

⤢ External intercostal muscle

⤢ Internal intercostal muscle

⤢ Innermost intercostal muscle

⤢ Pleura

Costal cartilages

Composed of hyaline cartilage and form multiple joints.

Sternocostal joints 1st rib to sternum is a fibrocartilagenous joint whereas 2nd to 7th are synovial

Interchondral joints Synovial joints; form mostly between the costal cartilages of the 'false ribs'

Muscles

Anterior chest wall consists of three muscles:

Pectoralis major

⤢ **Originates** from medial half of clavicle, sternum, and costal cartilages

⤢ **Inserts** lateral lip of intertubercular groove

⤢ **Acts** to adduct, flex, and medially rotate arm

⤢ **Innervation:** medial and lateral pectoral nerves

Pectoralis minor

⤢ Runs from 3rd–5th ribs to coracoid process

⤢ Is invested in the clavipectoral fascia

Subclavius

⤢ Runs from 1st rib to clavicle

Intercostal space

Between adjacent ribs; contains intercostal muscles.

External intercostals Run downwards and forward from rib above to below, act to move ribs superiorly

Internal intercostals Downwards and backwards from sternum to angle of rib, act to move ribs inferiorly

Innermost intercostals Move ribs inferiorly

Neurovascular bundles runs in costal groove through plane between inner two muscles.

Neurovascular contents:

⤢ Superior   Artery

             Vein

⤢ Inferior   Nerve

This makes the nerve most at risk of injury

Arterial supply

Comes via the anterior and posterior intercostal vessels which run in subcostal grooves.

Anterior intercostal arteries

1st to 6th	Derive from the internal thoracic artery
7th to 9th	From musculophrenic artery (terminal branch of the internal thoracic artery)

Posterior intercostal arteries

1st and 2nd	From superior intercostal branch of the costocervical trunk, a branch of subclavian artery
3rd to 11th	Branches of thoracic aorta

Venous drainage

Anterior intercostal veins

Both:

⤢ Anastomose with posterior veins

⤢ Drain into the internal thoracic and musculophrenic veins

Left-sided posterior intercostal veins

⤢ Upper veins converge to form left superior intercostal draining into brachiocephalic vein

⤢ Lower veins drain into hemiazygos system

Right-sided posterior intercostal veins

⤢ Upper vein drains directly into brachiocephalic

⤢ 2nd + 3rd form right superior intercostal which drains into azygos

⤢ Lower veins drain into the azygos system

2.2 Breast anatomy

Breast lies on pectoralis major and serratus anterior

Extends from:

⤢ 2nd to 6th rib

⤢ Sternum to midaxillary line

Remember, the 'tail' can extend into axillary apex.

Structure

⤢ 15–20 lobules of glandular tissue

⤢ Lactiferous duct from each lobe; open independently at the nipple

⤢ Fibrous septa (ligaments of Cooper) separate each lobule, and tension on these in breast carcinoma can lead to 'skin puckering'

⤢ Tissue present in men but functionless

Blood supply

⤢ Perforating branches of the internal thoracic artery

⤢ Branches of the axillary artery through breast; superior thoracic, lateral thoracic, subscapular, and thoracoacromial arteries

⤢ Perforators of the 2nd to 4th intercostal arteries

Lymph drainage
- Medial part to the intermammary nodes
- Lateral part to the axillary nodes

Innervation
- Via anterior and lateral branches of the 4th to 6th intercostal nerves

2.3 Abdominal wall

> The abdominal wall is comprised of layers of muscles and fascia. It is a subject introduced in examinations either by asking which layers are traversed at a given point by an incision or penetrating wound, or by questions about the inguinal region or rectus sheath.

You must be able to discuss the layers of the abdominal wall:
- Skin
- Superficial layer (Camper's fascia)
- Subcutaneous fat
- Deeper fibrous layer (Scarpa's fascia)
- External oblique
- Internal oblique
- Transverses abdominis
- Transveralis fascia
- Extraperitoneal fat
- Peritoneum

Muscular components
These muscles are divided into anterolateral and posterior compartments. The anterolateral group contain three lateral muscles whose aponeurosis forms the rectus sheath, in which the two anterior/vertical muscles are contained.

> **Midline incision**
> - Made through linea alba
> - Linea alba is broad above umbilicus, narrower below
> - This incision allows the surgeon a 'bloodless' field

The superior boundaries of the abdominal wall are the 7th to 10th costal cartilages and xiphoid process. The inferior boundary is the inguinal ligament, iliac crests, and the pubis.

External oblique
Fibres	Run downwards and forwards
Origin	Outer surface of lower eight ribs
Insertion	Pubic tubercle, iliac crest, and linea alba
Lower border	Forms inguinal ligament

Internal oblique
Fibres	Run upwards and forwards
Origin	Thoracolumbar fascia, iliac crest and inguinal ligament
Insertion	Inferior four ribs, linea alba, pubic crest

Transversus abdominis

Fibres Run transversely

Origin Thoracolumbar fascia, iliac crest, inguinal ligament, lower six costal cartilages

Insertion Linea alba and pubic crest

Rectus abdominis

Origin Anterior of 5th, 6th, and 7th costal cartilages

Insertion Pubic crest, tubercle, and symphysis

Linea semilunaris Represents the lateral border of the rectus abdominis

---

Composition of rectus sheath

↗ Superior to costal cartilage:
  - ◆ Anterior: external oblique aponeurosis
  - ◆ Posterior: no sheath

↗ Above arcuate line:
  - ◆ Anterior: external oblique and half of internal oblique aponeurosis
  - ◆ Posterior: Half of internal oblique and tranversus abdominis aponeurosis

↗ Below arcuate line:
  - ◆ Anterior: aponeurosis of all three muscles
  - ◆ Posterior: no sheath, transversalis fascia

Pyramidalis

Origin Pubic symphysis

Insertion Linea alba

Rectus sheath

↗ Composition varies along length but formed by aponeurosis of lateral muscles which fuse at the linea alba

↗ Has three tendinous intersections where anterior sheath attaches to the muscle itself

↗ Contains superior + inferior epigastric vessels, lower five ventral thoracic nerves, and lymphatics

Posterior wall muscles

Quadratus lumborum

Origin Iliolumbar ligament, iliac crest, and transverse process of L5 vertebra

Insertion Transverse process of L1–L4 and 12th rib

Psoas major

Origin Transverse processes of lumbar vertebra, vertebral bodies (T12–L5)

Insertion Lesser trochanter of femur

Iliacus

Origin Iliac fossa, sacroiliac and iliolumbar ligaments and sacrum

Insertion Lesser trochanter of femur

Blood supply

Abdominal wall has three main sources of blood:

- ↗ **Aorta,** via inferior phrenic, lumbar, intercostal, and subcostal arteries
- ↗ **Internal thoracic artery** via terminal branches: superior epigastric and musculophrenic arteries
- ↗ Branches of the **external iliac artery: inferior epigastric,** and **deep circumflex arteries**

Innervation

The anterior abdominal wall is supplied by the inferior six **thoracic nerves** (T7–T11), the **subcostal nerve** (T12), and the **iliohypogastric** and **ilioinguinal nerves** (L1).

These nerves run inferiorly in a parallel line to the ribs, in the plane between the internal oblique + transversus abdominis.

Lymph drainage

The lymphatic drainage of the abdominal wall is dependent on whether the structure is superficial or deep and if it is above or below the umbilicus:

Superficial Above umbilicus to axillary nodes and below to superficial inguinal nodes

Deep Follow path of arteries to para-aortic nodes

2.4 Inguinal canal

The inguinal canal represents the passage taken by the testes and cord during development from the abdomen to scrotum.

The inguinal canal is 4 cm long and passes downwards and medially from the deep (internal) ring to superficial (external) ring. It contains the **spermatic cord** (**round ligament** in the female) and the ilioinguinal nerve (L1).

Rings

Deep ring

- ↗ Opening in the transversalis fascia
- ↗ Lies halfway between the anterior superior iliac spine (ASIS) and pubic tubercle (midpoint of the inguinal ligament)
- ↗ Inferior epigastric vessels lie medially

Superficial ring

- ↗ Triangular defect in the external oblique aponeurosis
- ↗ Lies above and medial to pubic tubercle

Walls

Anterior External oblique (internal oblique lateral third)

Posterior Transversalis fascia (lateral part) conjoint tendon medially (common insertion of internal oblique and transversalis into pectineal line)

Superiorly Internal oblique

Inferiorly Inguinal ligament

2.5 Spermatic cord

The spermatic cord is the main structure transmitted through the inguinal canal. Its structure and contents are summarized by the 'rule of threes'

Rule of threes

Three layers

- ↗ External spermatic fascia (from external oblique aponeurosis)
- ↗ Cremasteric fascia (from the internal oblique aponeurosis)
- ↗ Internal spermatic fascia (from the transversalis fascia)

Three arteries

- ↗ Testicular artery
- ↗ Cremasteric artery
- ↗ Artery to the vas

Three nerves

- ↗ Genito-femoral
- ↗ Sympathetic fibres
- ↗ Ilioinguinal nerve (on the cord, not within)

Three other structures

- ↗ Vas deferens/round ligament
- ↗ Pampiniform plexus
- ↗ Lymphatics

Chapter 3 Heart and great vessels

A typical situation in the MRCS examination would be to have a heart opened with pins in any of the structures below. Easy marks would be to identify chambers/valves. Harder points would be for structures such as fossa ovalis.

3.1 Heart structure

Pericardium

↗ Outer fibrous layer which fuses with the roots of the great vessels

↗ Inner serous layer consisting of a parietal and a visceral layer (pericardial fluid between the parietal and visceral layers)

↗ Blood supply from pericardiophrenic branches of the internal thoracic artery

↗ Nerve supply from the phrenic nerve

Structures of note within the heart chambers

Right atrium (RA)

Sulcus terminalis	Vertical groove on the outer aspect of the RA
Crista terminalis	Muscular ridge on the inner aspect of the RA separating the smooth surface and the musculi pectinati
Fossa ovalis	Depression in the atrial septum (site of the foramen ovalis)

Right ventricle (RV)

Chordae tendinae	Attached to edges of the valve cusps and are themselves attached to the papillary wall muscles
Trabeculae carnae	Muscular bundles found within the ventricular wall
Moderator band	Contains the right branch of the atrioventricular bundle

3.2 Heart vasculature

Right coronary artery

↗ Supplies sinoatrial (SA) node in 60%

↗ Arises from the aortic sinus

↗ Branches

• Marginal

• Posterior interventricular branch

Left coronary artery

↗ Supplies SA node in 40%

↗ Arises from the aortic sinus

↗ Branches

• Anterior interventricular branch

• Posterior interventricular branch

Venous drainage

Veins accompanying the coronary arteries drain into the RA via the coronary sinus.

Venae cordis minimi	Small veins draining directly into the RA

3.3 Thoracic vasculature

Thoracic aorta

The **ascending aorta** arises from the aortic vestibule behind the infundibulum of the right ventricle and the pulmonary trunk. It is continuous with the **aortic arch**, which lies posterior to the lower half of the manubrium and arches from front to back over the left main bronchus.

The **descending thoracic aorta** is continuous with the arch and begins at the lower border of the body of T4. It enters the diaphragm beneath the median arcuate ligament of the diaphragm at the level of T12.

Branches of the ascending aorta

* Left and right coronary arteries

Branches of the aortic arch

* Brachiocephalic artery: bifurcates into the right subclavian and right common carotid arteries posterior to the right sternoclavicular joint
* Left common carotid
* Left subclavian
* Thyroid ima

Branches of the descending aorta

* Oesophageal
* Bronchial
* Mediastinal
* Posterior intercostals
* Subcostal

Chapter 4 Lungs and diaphragm

You will need to be comfortable in describing the anatomy of the lungs and diaphragm. Surface anatomy regularly comes up in a station with a live model, and cross-sectional imaging may be used to introduce the topic in a manned station.

4.1 Pleura

The thorax contains two pleural cavities separated by the **mediastinum**. During development the lung grows out of the mediastinum incorporating the pleura as its lining. The pleura are thin fibrous membranes consisting of parietal and visceral layers with a **'potential' pleural space** between.

In pathological states the pleural space can be filled with air, fluid, blood, or pus.

The lung does not fill the entire pleural space; the unoccupied space is important for allowing full lung expansion in deep inspiration. This space described as the **costodiaphragmatic** and **costomediastinal recesses.**

Parietal pleura

Described according to the part of thoracic wall it is in contact with; **costal, diaphragmatic, mediastinal,** and **cervical** parts.

Costal part	innervated by the **intercostal nerves**
Diaphragmatic part	innervated by the **phrenic nerve**
Mediastinal part	innervated by the **phrenic nerve**

Visceral pleura

* Adherent to lung surfaces and extends into the lung fissures
* Supplied by **autonomic nerve** fibres sensate to stretch only
* Continuous at the hilum with the parietal pleura

4.2 Lungs

The two lungs sit on either side of the mediastinum in completely separate pleural cavities. The right lung is slightly larger and has an additional third lobe.

The **lung root carries** important structures between the mediastinum and the lung, entering at the **hilum:**

* Pulmonary artery
* Two pulmonary veins
* Main bronchus
* Bronchial vessels
* Pulmonary nerve plexus
* Lymphatics

The **pulmonary ligament** is an inferior extension of the pleura at the hilum allowing for movement during inspiration.

Usual orientation at the hilum

* Pulmonary artery sits superiorly
* Pulmonary veins inferiorly
* Bronchus posteriorly

The lung lobes are further subdivided into the **bronchopulmonary segments.** These are the smallest functionally independent lung units. **Each segment has its own segmental bronchus and branch of pulmonary artery.** Surgically this is important as a segment can be resected without any effect on the rest of the lung.

Right lung

There are three lobes and two fissures:

Oblique fissure   Separates the inferior from the superior and middle lobes

Horizontal fissure   Separates the superior and middle lobes

Medially the right lung is in contact with; the heart, inferior vena cava (IVC), superior vena cava (SVC), azygos vein, and oesophagus.

> **Surface markings**
> * **Horizontal fissure**—Runs from the 4th intercostal space at the sternum and meets the oblique fissure as it crosses the 5th rib
> * **Oblique fissure**—Runs in a curved line from the spinous process of T4 to the 5th intercostal space laterally before following the 6th rib anteriorly

Left lung

* Two lobes which are separated by the oblique fissure
* Medial relations of the left lung include the heart, aortic arch, and oesophagus
* Indented by the heart on its medial surface
  * The **lingula** is a cuff of lung tissue which overlies this indentation and forms part of the superior lobe

4.3 Bronchial tree

Trachea

* Start of the 'bronchial tree' at the level of cricoid cartilage (C6) as a continuation of the larynx
* 10 cm long and 2 cm in diameter
* Consists of 15–20 C-shaped hyaline cartilages and bifurcates at T4/5 into the two main bronchi

Bronchi

* Main bronchi divide into lobar bronchi distal to the pulmonary root; an exception is the lobar bronchus to the right superior lobe which originates before
* Lobar bronchi then further divide into segmental bronchi which supply individual bronchopulmonary segments

Blood supply

* Deoxygenated blood is carried to the lungs by the pulmonary trunk which **bifurcates at T4/5** to the right and left pulmonary arteries
* After oxygenation blood is transported back to the left atrium through bilateral superior and inferior pulmonary veins
* The bronchial arteries originate from the **thoracic aorta** and the bronchial veins drain either into the pulmonary veins or the **azygos system**

Lymphatics

* Lymph drainage is initially to the **bronchopulmonary nodes** at the lung hilar
* Drainage continues to the tracheobronchial nodes around the carina and then the bronchomediastinal trunks
* Lymph enters the venous system through either the right lymphatic duct or thoracic duct on the left

4.4 Diaphragm

Function

The diaphragm plays a central role in inspiration and is aided by the accessory respiratory muscles: external intercostals, **scalene and sternocleidomastoid** muscles

Expansion occurs in three directions:

↗ **Vertical**: increased by contraction of the diaphragm

↗ **AP**: movement of sternum relative to the ribs and can be visualized as a 'pump handle'

↗ **Lateral**: movement of the ribs up and outwards which can be visualized by a 'bucket handle'

The diaphragm is a domed musculotendinous sheet that acts as a partition between the thoracic and abdominal cavities. It runs superiorly from its **posterior attachment at T12** to the xiphoid process anteriorly. It has a **central tendon** and peripheral muscular parts.

Paralysis of the diaphragm is recognized by elevation of the diaphragm and paradoxical movement.

Vertebral diaphragm

↗ Originates from crura and arcuate ligaments

↗ Right crus originates from L1–3 vertebra

↗ Left crus from L1 and L2 vertebra

↗ Medial arcuate ligament from psoas major fascia

↗ Lateral arcuate ligament from quadratus lumborum fascia

Costal and sternal diaphragm

↗ Attached to the inner aspect of the lower six ribs and the sternal part to the xiphoid process

Diaphragm openings

T8 Vena cava and right phrenic nerve

T10 Oesophagus, vagus nerve, oesophageal branches of left gastric vessels, and lymphatics

T12 Aorta, azygos vein, and thoracic duct

Blood supply

Branches of the internal thoracic artery:

↗ Pericardiophrenic artery

↗ Musculophrenic artery

↗ Branches of the aorta

↗ Superior phrenic artery

↗ Inferior phrenic artery

↗ Lower five intercostal arteries

Venous drainage typically mirrors that of the arterial supply draining into the azygos system, brachio-cephalic veins, or IVC.

Innervation

The diaphragm is innervated by the two **phrenic nerves** which originate from C3, C4, and C5.

Remember: C3, 4, and 5, keep you alive!

The phrenic nerves pass down from the neck, through the superior thoracic aperture, anterior to the lung roots before supplying the diaphragm.

Diaphragmatic hernia

↗ Can be **congenital**:

- **Bochdalek's**, occurring posteriorly
- **Morgagni's**, occurring at the junction between the costal cartilages and xiphoid process

↗ Or **acquired**:

- **Sliding hiatus hernia** where oesophagogastric junction slides up into the thorax
- **Rolling hiatus hernia** when part of the stomach in the thorax but junction remains in abdomen

Chapter 5 **Oesophagus and stomach**

5.1 Oesophagus

The oesophagus descends through the root of the neck and traverses the thoracic inlet behind the trachea lying in front of the upper four thoracic vertebrae. It continues into the posterior mediastinum in front of the 5th thoracic vertebrae accompanied by the right and left vagus nerves. It passes through the diaphragm at the level of T10.

Structure

- Inner mucosa of stratified squamous epithelium
- Submucosal layer
- Double muscular layer—longitudinal outer layer and circular inner layer (striated muscle in upper 2/3 and smooth muscle lower 1/3)
- Outer layer of areolar tissue

Blood supply

- Inferior thyroid arteries
- Descending thoracic aorta
- Left gastric artery

Venous drainage

- Lower oesophagus into the azygous system via the left gastric vein
- Upper oesophagus via the braciocephalic veins

Innervation

- Sensory and parasympathetic motor fibres via the vagus nerves and their recurrent laryngeal branches

5.2 Stomach

The stomach lies in the upper part of the abdomen beneath the left dome of the diaphragm. It is classically described as having three parts—fundus, body, and antrum. It has anterior and posterior surfaces joined by a lesser and greater curvature. A notch (**incisura angularis**) may be present on the lesser curve near the pyloric region. A well-developed smooth muscle coat which is thickened around the pyloric region forms the **pyloric sphincter**.

Arterial supply

- Left gastric artery
- Right gastric artery
- Right gastroepiploic artery
- Left gastroepiploic artery
- Short gastric artery

Gastric arterial supply is a favoured MRCS examination topic. All vessels originate from the **coeliac trunk (T12)** which gives rise to the hepatic artery (right gastric), gastroduodenal artery (right gastroepiploic), and splenic artery (short gastric and left epiploic artery).

Venous drainage

Gastric veins accompany their arteries and drain into the portal venous system:

- The portal vein receives the right and left gastric veins
- The splenic vein receives the short gastric and left gastroepiploic veins
- The right gastroepiploic vein enters the superior mesenteric vein

Innervation

- The anterior vagal trunk (predominantly derived from the left vagus) gives branches to the anterior surface of the stomach and pyloric region
- The posterior vagal trunk (predominantly derived from the right vagus) gives branches to the posterior surface and coeliac plexus

Chapter 6 Liver, pancreas, and biliary system

6.1 Liver

The liver is a favourite for prosection stations and you should be confident describing its anatomy. Conditions affecting these systems will be in the MRCS examination, and knowledge of the anatomy is vital to show understanding of the topic.

The liver is the largest internal organ and embryologically develops from the foregut. It is located mainly in the right hypochondrium but can extend into the epigastrium and left hypochondrium.

You should be able to describe its functions, surfaces, ligaments, and lobes in the examination.

Functions

- Metabolism of glucose: glycogenesis, glycogenolysis, and gluconeogenesis
- Metabolism of lipids: production of free fatty acids and synthesis of cholesterol
- Metabolism of protein: breakdown to ammonia, synthesis of clotting factors and albumin
- Vitamins: activation of D and storage of A, D, E, K, and B_{12}
- Detoxification of drugs, toxins, and hormones
- Haematopoiesis in children (occasionally adults)

Surfaces

The liver has three borders (superior, inferior, lateral) and two surfaces:

Diaphragmatic surface
- In contact with the diaphragm in anterior, superior, and posterior directions
- Between the liver and the diaphragm there are potential gaps, described as the **subphrenic** and **hepatorenal recesses**, where pathological fluid may collect

Visceral surface
- Postero-inferior direction, covered by visceral peritoneum
- In contact with five organs: stomach, duodenum, gallbladder, colon, and right kidney

Be able to recognize and describe the H-shaped structure on the visceral surface of the liver.

An H-shaped configuration can be seen on the surface where the vertical lines are made up anteriorly on the right by the gallbladder fossa and the left by the ligamentum teres, posteriorly on the right by the bed of the IVC and the left by the ligamentum venosum. The horizontal line represents the **porta hepatis**, which is the site of transit of the hepatic arteries, portal vein, and hepatic ducts.

When asked to orientate the portal triad, think '**P**' and '**LARD**':
- **Portal vein is posterior**
- **Left is Artery**
- **Right is Duct**

Ligaments

Falciform ligament	Attaches the liver to the anterior abdominal wall separating the liver anatomically into right and left lobes
Anterior and posterior coronary ligaments	Reflections of the peritoneum from the diaphragmatic surface
Right and left triangular ligaments	Extensions of the coronary ligament that help delineate the bare area

Ligamentum teres	Fetal remnant of the left umbilical vein whose function was to bring blood from placenta to fetus
Ligamentum venosum	Fetal remnant of the ductus venosus which acted to shunt oxygenated blood past the liver to the IVC
Hepatoduodenal ligament	The 'free edge of lesser omentum' runs between the liver and duodenum and contains the common hepatic artery, portal vein, and common bile duct

The **'bare area'** is the only part of the liver not covered by visceral peritoneum and is on the diaphragmatic surface.

Lobes

The lobes of the liver can be described functionally or anatomically.

The liver is **anatomically** divided into right and left lobes by the falciform ligament (anteriorly). Infero-posteriorly the ligamentum venosum and teres help to identify the **caudate** and **quadrate lobes**, with the caudate lobe bordered by ligamentum venosum and the IVC and the quadrate lobe by ligamentum teres and the gallbladder fossa.

However, the liver is preferably divided **functionally** according to its blood supply to different lobes/segments. The functional right and left lobes can be illustrated by drawing a vertical line through the IVC and gallbladder bed. This can be extended to divide the liver into **eight segments** according to the branches of the **portal vein** and **hepatic artery**. These segments become surgically important when performing hepatic resections.

Blood supply and drainage

The liver has a dual blood supply. The **portal vein** supplies around 70% of blood and is formed by the union of **superior mesenteric** and **splenic veins** posterior to the pancreatic neck at level of transpyloric plane.

The left and **right hepatic arteries** supply the rest and originate from the coeliac artery, via the **common hepatic artery**.

The liver usually drains via three **hepatic veins** directly into the IVC just below the level of the diaphragm.

There are four **portosystemic shunts**:
↗ Left gastric veins to oesophageal veins
↗ Superior rectal to middle and inferior rectal veins
↗ Paraumbilical to epigastric veins on the anterior abdominal wall
↗ Retroperitoneally branches of splenic and pancreatic veins to left renal vein

6.2 Gallbladder

Function

↗ To receive, concentrate, store, and secrete bile into the duodenum
↗ The secretion of bile is primarily under hormonal control, with **cholecystokinin** being released in response to the presence of fat in the duodenum

> During surgery, bleeding can by controlled by **Pringle's manoeuvre:**
> ↗ Hepatic artery is compressed by finger and thumb as it runs in the epiploic foramen

Anatomy
↗ 7–10 cm long; sits adherent to the visceral surface of the right lobe of the liver

↗ Has a fundus, body, and neck

↗ Pathological dilatation just proximal to the gallbladder neck is termed **Hartmann's pouch**

Blood supply
↗ Mostly via the cystic artery (branch of the right hepatic artery)

↗ Also via branches of hepatic artery from its fossa

↗ There is no cystic vein and instead venous drainage occurs through the gallbladder bed

> Complications of gallstones include biliary colic, cholecystitis, obstructive jaundice, pancreatitis, cholangitis, and gallstone ileus.

6.3 Biliary system

The biliary system begins in the liver where ducts congregate to form the right and left hepatic ducts. These unite to form the common hepatic duct which runs in the **porta hepatis.**

> **Calot's triangle**
> ↗ Contains the cystic artery
> ↗ Its boundaries are:
> - ◆ Superiorly: liver
> - ◆ Inferiorly: cystic duct
> - ◆ Medially: common hepatic duct

The **cystic duct**, which drains the gallbladder, joins this common hepatic duct to form the **common bile duct.** The common bile duct runs in the free edge of the lesser omentum and passes posterior to the duodenum where it is usually joined by the main pancreatic duct and drains into the second part of the duodenum at the **ampulla of Vater.**

6.4 Pancreas

Function
Exocrine function   To break down proteins, fats, and carbohydrates so that they can be absorbed

Endocrine function To regulate glucose levels through the secretion of glucagon and insulin

> **Pancreatitis**
> ↗ Results from activation of exocrine proenzymes and autodigestion of the organ
> ↗ Common causes are gallstones and ethanol
> ↗ **Glasgow** and **Ranson** systems estimate severity

Position
↗ The gland is mostly retroperitoneal and extends across the posterior abdominal wall at the transpyloric plane

↗ The splenic artery runs at its superior margin and the splenic vein posteriorly which can results in splenic vein thrombosis in patients with pancreatitis

↗ Anteriorly the pancreas is situated behind the stomach with the lesser sac between. Pathological fluid can accumulate in this sac, e.g. in perforated gastric ulcer or pancreatitis

Posterior relations of the pancreas

These include:

↗ Superior mesenteric vessels

↗ IVC

↗ Aorta

↗ Left kidney and adrenal gland

Anatomy

↗ Anatomical parts are described as the head, neck, body, tail, and uncinate process

↗ The head is located adjacent to the duodenum, the tail extends towards the spleen, and these two parts are intraperitoneal

↗ The main duct **(duct of Wirsung)** extends from the tail to the head before joining the bile duct and draining into the duodenum

↗ The accessory duct **(duct of Santorini)** runs from the uncinate process and empties above the main duct into the duodenum

Surgical removal of the pancreas necessitates removal of the duodenum as they share a blood supply.

Blood supply

Coeliac trunk	• Anterior and posterior superior pancreaticoduodenal artery • Splenic artery branches
Superior mesenteric artery (SMA)	Anterior and posterior inferior pancreaticoduodenal arteries

Chapter 7 **Small and large intestines**

The bowel has many common pathologies and an understanding of its anatomy will help you approach and answer questions in the MRCS examination.

7.1 Overview

As a result of the way the intestines develop it is typically described in terms of the foregut, midgut, and hindgut:

Foregut

↗ From oropharynx to 2nd part of the duodenum

↗ Supplied by coeliac trunk (T12)

Midgut

↗ From 2nd part of the duodenum to distal third of the transverse colon

↗ Supplied by SMA (L1)

Hindgut

↗ From distal third of the transverse colon to the anus

↗ Supplied by inferior mesenteric artery (L3)

The basic structure of the alimentary tract is made up of layers (from interior outwards):

↗ Mucosa

↗ Muscularis mucosa

↗ Submucosa

↗ Muscle

↗ Serosa

7.2 Small intestine

The small intestine has an average length of 6 m and extends from the pyloric sphincter to the ileocaecal junction. It is suspended from the posterior abdominal wall on the 'mesentery of the small intestine' and has three parts; the duodenum, jejunum, and ileum.

Duodenum

The duodenum is a C-shaped structure surrounding the head of the pancreas. It is around 25 cm long and has four parts:

Superior (5 cm)

↗ Runs from pylorus to the right side of L1

↗ Is the only intraperitoneal part

↗ Posterior relations are common bile duct, portal vein, and gastroduodenal artery

Descending (7 cm)

↗ Runs inferiorly from level of L1 to L2

↗ Common bile duct and major and accessory pancreatic ducts enter here

Inferior (10 cm)

↗ Longest section passing in front of IVC and aorta to the left side of L3

Ascending (2.5 cm)

↗ Passes upwards to the level of L2 and terminates at the duodenojejunal flexure which is supported by the ligament of Treitz, a peritoneal fold

Blood supply

Via coeliac arteries and SMA:

Coeliac arteries Anterior and posterior superior pancreaticoduodenal arteries

SMA Anterior and posterior inferior pancreaticoduodenal arteries

> Posterior duodenal ulcers can be complicated by erosion of the gastroduodenal artery causing haemorrhage.

Jejunum and ileum

These parts form most of the length of the small intestine. In both, the mucosa has numerous folds called **plicae circulares**.

Blood supply is via the jejunal and ileal arteries branches of the SMA. These unite to form arterial arcades which form the straight vasa recta which pass to the intestine

> **Differences between ileum and jejunum**
> - Jejunum forms two-fifths and ileum three-fifths of the small intestines
> - Jejunum has a thicker wall and larger diameter
> - Jejunum is dark red and ileum paler pink
> - Jejunum typically lies centrally or in the left upper quadrant; ileum lies in the right lower quadrant
> - Jejunum has less prominent arterial arcades and longer vasa recta
> - Ileum has thicker mesentery and has Peyer's patches

7.3 Large intestine

The large intestine extends from the distal ileum to the anus and functions to absorb fluid and salts. It is 1.5 m long and is described in eight parts: caecum, appendix, ascending colon, transverse colon, descending colon, sigmoid colon, rectum, and anal canal.

The typical features of the large bowel include:

- Larger diameter
- Appendices epiploicae
- Taenia coli—three bands of longitudinal muscles
- Haustra—sacculation caused by contraction of taenia coli

> **Meckel's diverticulum** is a congenital remnant of vitelline duct occurring in 2% of the population.

Caecum

The caecum is an intraperitoneal structure which is usually found in the right iliac fossa. It is a continuation of the ileum which enters at an oblique angle and has two ileocaecal folds extending into the caecum that form the ileocaecal sphincter.

Blood supply is via anterior and posterior caecal arteries from the ileocolic branches of the SMA

> - The caecum has the largest diameter (7–9 cm) and so is most likely site of colonic **perforation**
> - Sigmoid colon is the narrowest section and so is the most likely site of **obstruction**

Appendix

The appendix is a narrow blind-ended tube attached to the posteromedial wall of the caecum. It is suspended from the terminal ileum by the mesoappendix which contains the appendicular vessels.

Its position is highly variable and can be described as retrocaecal (commonest), pelvic, subcaecal, or preileal. However, the position of its base is consistent on the caecum where the three bands of the taenia coli converge.

Blood supply via the appendicular artery from the ileocolic branches of the SMA.

Colon

Caecum continues superiorly as the **ascending colon** to the hepatic flexure. It then crosses the abdomen as the **transverse colon** to the splenic flexure and continues inferiorly as the **descending** and then **sigmoid colon**.

The ascending and descending colon are retroperitoneal, whereas the transverse and sigmoid parts have mesenteries and are thus intraperitoneal.

Important spaces exist between the ascending and descending colon and the posterolateral abdominal wall. These are known as the **right and left paracolic gutters** respectively and can be sites for the collection of pathological fluid.

> **Classic symptoms of large-bowel obstruction**
> ↗ Absolute constipation
> ↗ Vomiting
> ↗ Abdominal distension
> ↗ Colicky pain
>
> **Common causes:**
> ↗ Tumour
> ↗ Hernia
> ↗ Diverticular disease

Blood supply

Through both the SMA and the inferior mesenteric artery (IMA):

SMA
- Colic branch of ileocolic artery
- Right colic artery
- Middle colic artery

IMA
- Left colic artery
- Sigmoid arteries

The **marginal artery of Drummond** connects the SMA and IMA arteries described above.

> A 'watershed' area occurs at the splenic flexure which lies between the areas supplied by superior and inferior mesenteric arteries.

Rectum

The rectum is a retroperitoneal structure, 2 cm long, which is a continuation of the sigmoid colon at the level of S3 and inferiorly continues at the anal canal.

The taenia coli of the colon form a continuous outer longitudinal layer of smooth muscle over the rectum. The peritoneal coverings vary according to rectal level:

Upper third   Extraperitoneal posteriorly

Middle third   Extraperitoneal posteriorly and laterally

Lower third	Completely extraperitoneal
Posterior relations	Sacrum, coccyx, sacral nerves
Anterior relations	Pouch of Douglas, small intestine, bladder, prostate, vagina, and uterus
Lateral relations	Levator ani

> The pouch of Douglas is the space between the rectum and bladder or uterus.

Blood supply
- Superior rectal artery from IMA
- Internal iliac artery
- Middle rectal artery
- Inferior rectal artery

Anal canal

The anal canal is is 4 cm long and runs from the rectum to anal orifice.

A boundary exists between the endoderm and ectoderm parts which have differing features:

Upper half (endoderm)
- **Has columnar epithelium**
- Supplied by superior rectal vessels
- Drains to lumbar nodes

Lower half (ectoderm)
- **Has squamous epithelium**
- Supplied by middle and inferior rectal vessels
- Drains to inguinal nodes

Venous drainage

The intestines and associated structures drain via the portal system to the liver.

↗ The **inferior mesenteric vein** drains the hindgut before joining with the splenic vein

↗ The **superior mesenteric vein** drains the midgut and unites with the splenic vein to form the portal vein behind neck of pancreas at level of transpyloric plane

If the portal system becomes blocked, blood may return to the heart via four potential portosystemic shunts.

Lymph drainage

Lymph drainage occurs along the mesentery to nodes near the origin of the coeliac, superior mesenteric and inferior mesenteric arteries. The lymph then drains superiorly through the cisterna chyli.

Chapter 8 **Urinary system**

The anatomy and function of the renal tract is a common topic in the MRCS examination, especially in the prosection stations. You should therefore be confident identifying and then describing the key elements. As there are lots of similar-looking structures in the abdomen and pelvis, practise following them up and down to help identify them.

8.1 Kidneys

Function

The kidney has six main functions:

* Fluid balance
* Acid–base balance
* Maintenance of electrolytes (importantly potassium)
* Excreting waste products
* Production of erythropoietin and renin
* Activation of vitamin D

Anatomy

The kidneys consist of an inner medulla and outer cortex. They lie retroperitoneally on the posterior abdominal wall with the superior pole below the 12th rib and the inferior pole at the level of L3. Because of the position of the liver, the right kidney lies slightly lower than the left.

Each kidney is 10–12 cm in size and surrounded by a fibrous capsule; outside this lies perinephric fat contained within **Gerota's fascia**.

The **renal hilum** is located on the medial aspect of each kidney at the transpyloric level. This is the point of transit for vessels. Their layout here is a common examination question and can be recalled by the acronym 'VAP-AP' (see box).

> **Renal hilum—'VAP-AP'** (vein, artery, pelvis, anterior to posterior):
> * Renal vein anteriorly
> * Renal artery
> * Renal pelvis posteriorly

The urine produced by the kidney drains through minor calices into major calices before joining to form the renal pelvis which continues inferiorly as the ureter.

> Transplant patients can be found in clinical examinations, so remember the procedure is performed extraperitoneally. The organ is sited in the left or right iliac fossa and connected to the external iliac vessels.

Relations

Right kidney

From superior to inferior:

Anterior   Adrenal gland, liver, duodenum, colon, small intestine

Posterior   Diaphragm, 12th rib, three muscles (psoas major, quadratus lumborum and tranversus abdominis), and three nerves (subcostal, iliohypogastric, ilioinguinal)

Left kidney

From superior to inferior:

Anterior   Adrenal gland, stomach, spleen, pancreas, colon, small intestines

Posterior   Same as right kidney

> **Remember:** the aorta sits on the left side, meaning the right renal artery is longer and runs posterior to the IVC, whereas the left renal vein is longer and runs anterior to the aorta.

Blood supply and lymphatics

The kidneys are supplied by the renal arteries arising from the aorta at L2. Accessory renal arteries are common.

At the hilum the renal artery divides into five segmental arteries, each supplying a separate resectable segment before further dividing within the kidney itself.

Blood is transported back to the IVC via the renal vein and the lymph drains into the para-aortic nodes.

8.2 Ureters

The ureter is a 20–30 cm muscular tube lined by transitional epithelium. It functions to transport urine from the kidney to the bladder. It is retroperitoneal throughout its course and is closely adherent to the parietal peritoneum.

> **Remember:** there is more than one common structure that is 20–30 cm in length:
> ↗ Ureter
> ↗ Oesophagus
> ↗ Duodenum

Course

From the renal pelvis the ureters pass along the medial border of psoas major, anterior to the transverse processes of L2–L5. They cross the common iliac bifurcation anterior to the sacroiliac joint and pass down the lateral pelvic wall. At the level of the ischial spines the ureters turn forward and medially, entering the bladder obliquely and thus helping prevent reflux.

In the male pelvis the vas deferens passes anteriorly, whereas in the female the ureter passes posterior to the uterine vessels.

> Typically three narrowings of the ureter:
> ↗ Ureteropelvic junction
> ↗ As the ureter crosses pelvic brim
> ↗ Vesicoureteric junction

Blood supply

Upper third   By the renal arteries
Middle third   From branches of the aorta and gonadal arteries
Inferior third   Branches from internal iliac and inferior vesical artery

> During surgical procedures the ureter is identified by its 'vermicular' movements when touched.

8.3 Adrenal glands

Anatomy

The adrenal glands sit on the superomedial aspect of each kidney, surrounded by perinephric fat within the renal fascia.

The adrenal **medulla** is made up of nervous tissue derived from neural crest cells. These chromaffin cells act as postganglionic neurons, secreting noradrenaline and adrenaline in response to preganglionic stimulation.

> **Phaeochromocytoma** is a rare catecholamine-secreting tumour of chromaffin cells.
>
> **Remember:** before surgical intervention, both alpha and beta receptor blockade is required.

The adrenal cortex has three layers which secrete different hormones:

Zona glomerulosa   mineralocorticoids (e.g. aldosterone)

Zona fasciculate   glucocorticoids (e.g. cortisol)

Zona reticularis   inner layer, secreting androgens

Blood supply

↗ Superior adrenal artery branch of the inferior phrenic artery

↗ Middle adrenal artery direct branch from the aorta

↗ Inferior adrenal artery branch of the renal artery

Venous drainage usually occurs via a single vein, to the IVC on the right and to the renal vein on the left.

8.4 Bladder

The bladder functions to collect and store urine ready for micturition. It is lined by transitional epithelium and its wall contains the detrusor muscle.

Anatomy

Predominantly a pelvic organ in adults, the bladder can extend palpably into the abdomen when full. It is pyramidal in shape and has various parts:

↗ The apex projects anteriorly

↗ The base is angled posteroinferiorly and forms a triangular **trigone**.

• The ureters enter at the superior two corners of the trigone and the urethra leaves at the inferior corner

↗ The bladder neck is inferior and is held in position by the puboprostatic and pubovesical ligaments.

Relations

Anterior   Pubic symphysis and peritoneum if empty

Posterior   In males the rectum and seminal vesicles; in women the cervix and upper part of the vagina

Superior   Peritoneum and bowel

Inferior   Sits on the pelvic diaphragm and musculature

Lateral   Levator ani and obturator internus

> An empty bladder is covered both anteriorly and superiorly by peritoneum. When full this covering is just superiorly, and this allows safe suprapubic catheterization to be performed.

Blood supply and lymphatics

The superior and inferior vesical arteries supply the bladder and are branches of the internal iliac artery. The drainage of venous blood mirrors the arterial system and the lymph drains to the para-aortic nodes.

Innervation (autonomic)

Parasympathetic   • Contract detrusor muscle
• Inhibit internal sphincters

| Sympathetic | • Inhibit detrusor muscle |
| | • Stimulate sphincter |

> **Remember:** the external sphincter has striated muscle, is under voluntary control, and is supplied by the pudendal nerve.

8.5 Urethra

The urethra is lined by transitional epithelium and acts to transport urine out of the bladder. It differs between the sexes:

Women

The urethra is 4 cm long and follows a straight course. It passes through the pelvic floor and perineum, where it is surrounded by external urethral sphincters, before opening anterior to the vagina in the vestibule.

Men

The urethra is 20 cm long and its course is more complicated; its parts are described according to position:

Preprostatic	• Between bladder neck and prostate
	• Position of **internal urethral sphincters**
Prostatic	• As passes through prostate
Membranous	• Narrowest part
	• Surrounded by external sphincters
	• Urethra bends anteriorly as enters penis
Spongy	Contains a further inferior bend
	• Opens at the external urethral meatus

8.6 Scrotum and testes

Scrotal structure

The scrotum is a cutaneous sac that contains the testes, spermatic cord, and epididymis. The skin has a wrinkled appearance due to the adherent **dartos fascia**, has multiple sebaceous glands, and is marked by the longitudinal **medial raphe** vertically in the midline.

Scrotal layers

⤢ Scrotal skin

⤢ Dartos fascia (retracts testes)

⤢ External spermatic fascia continuation of external oblique

⤢ Cremasteric fascia continuation of internal oblique

⤢ Internal spermatic fascia continuation of tranversus abdominis

Testes

Overview

The main function of the testes is spermatogenesis, and for this reason during development they descend from the posterior abdominal wall through the inguinal canal to the scrotum where the temperature is nearly 3° cooler. They carry vessels, nerves, lymphatics, and the **ductus deferens** with them during this migration.

Anatomy

The testes consist of lobules containing **seminiferous tubules** that produce spermatozoa. These tubules unite to form the **rete testis** which drains into the epididymis.

The epididymis lies posterolateral to testes and transports sperm from the testes to the **ductus deferens.**

The testis has a surrounding thick capsule known as the **tunica albuginea.** External to this the testis is covered all but posteriorly by the **tunica vaginalis,** which is derived from the peritoneum.

Blood supply and lymphatics

Blood reaches the testes via the testicular artery which is a direct branch from the aorta and anastomoses with the **artery to the vas deferens.** The artery to the vas is a branch of the **inferior vesical artery,** and supplies the epididymis and vas deferens.

Blood drains via the **pampiniform plexus** to either IVC on the right side or the renal vein on the left. The testicular lymphatics drain to the **para-aortic nodes.**

> Radical orchidectomy is performed through an inguinal incision to prevent involvement of scrotal lymphatics.
>
> **Remember:** the lymph drainage of the scrotum and testes differs:
>
> ↗ Testes to para-aortic
>
> ↗ Scrotum to inguinal

8.7 Prostate

The prostate is approximately 3 cm long and 4 cm wide. It is described as having anterior, posterior, middle, and lateral lobes, and contains mainly glandular tissue. The ejaculatory ducts run through the prostate and open into the prostatic urethra. The prostatic urethral lumen contains a longitudinal midline fold known as the **urethral crest;** laterally at this point the prostatic ducts empty at the **prostatic sinus.**

Relations

Anteriorly	Pubic symphysis with retropubic space between
Superiorly	Base is in contact with the bladder
Posteriorly	Separated from the rectum by fascia of Denonvilliers
Inferiorly	Apex sits on the pelvic floor

Blood supply

Blood supply via the **inferior vesical artery** and venous drainage via a plexus either to the internal iliac vessels or the internal vertebral venous plexus.

> It is suggested that the commonly occurring spinal metastasis in prostate cancer is linked with the direct venous drainage to the prevertebral plexus.

Section 2 Pathology and Physiology

Chapter 9 Thoracic pathology

9.1 Valvular heart disease

Although heart auscultation and diagnosis of valvular disease is commonly seen as a medical problem, it can come up in a thoracic station in the MRCS examination and so at least a basic knowledge is required.

Mitral regurgitation

Mitral regurgitation is the commonest valvular lesion.

⤤ May present acutely with signs of congestive cardiac failure

⤤ Chronic regurgitation presents with:

- Exertional dyspnoea
- Orthopnoea

Causes

⤤ Mitral valve prolapse (due to rupture of chordae tendinae)

⤤ Rheumatic heart disease

⤤ Endocarditis

Clinical findings

⤤ Pansystolic murmur radiating to axilla

⤤ Displaced apex beat

⤤ Atrial fibrillation in 80%

Investigation

Chest radiograph (CXR)

Transthoracic or transoesophageal echocardiogram (TTE/TOE)

Mitral stenosis

Associated with rheumatic heart disease.

Clinical findings

⤤ Dyspnoea

⤤ Haemoptysis

⤤ Atrial fibrillation

⤤ Left parasternal heave

⤤ Tapping apex beat

⤤ Mid-diastolic murmur at apex

Investigations

⤤ CXR

⤤ TTE/TOE

Aortic stenosis

Associated with calcific degeneration, bicuspid valve, and rheumatic heart disease.

Clinical features

⤤ Angina, syncope, and dyspnoea

⤤ Slow rising, low volume pulse

⤤ Heaving apex beat

⤤ Ejection systolic murmur radiating to carotids

Investigations

Electrocardiogram (ECG)

CXR

TTE/TOE

Aortic regurgitation

Associated with rheumatic heart disease, endocarditis, aortic dissection, and connective tissue disorders (e.g. Marfan's).

Clinical features

⤤ Orthopnoea, fatigue, dyspnoea

⤤ Wide pulse pressure/collapsing 'water hammer pulse'

⤤ Early diastolic murmur

Associated signs

Austin Flint murmur	Mid-diastolic murmur
Quinke's sign	Nail bed pulsation
Corrigan's sign	Visible neck pulsation
De Musset's sign	Head nodding
Du Rozier's sign	Femoral diastolic murmur

Treatment

Medical optimization.

Patients who are symptomatic

Surgical treatment should be considered in all patients with valvular disease who are symptomatic.

Patients who are asymptomatic

Mitral regurgitation/aortic regurgitation

⤤ Patients who are asymptomatic but show signs on echocardiogram of worsening left ventricular systolic dysfunction (increasing dilatation of the ventricle and decreasing ejection fraction)

⤤ Treatment options are valve repair or valve replacement

Aortic stenosis/mitral stenosis

⤤ Patients with evidence of severe stenosis should be considered for surgical management even if asymptomatic

⤤ Valve area <1 cm^2 indicates severe stenosis

⤤ Treatment options are percutaneous balloon valvuloplasty, open valvotomy, and valve replacement

9.2 Pericardial effusion

There is normally approximately 20 mL of pericardial fluid within the pericardial space. A pericardial effusion is an abnormal accumulation of pericardial fluid. It may be acute or chronic.

Causes

⤤ Pericarditis

⤤ Congestive cardiac failure

⤢ Metastatic spread

⤢ Lymphoma

⤢ Leukaemia

⤢ Autoimmune disorders

Investigations

⤢ CXR

⤢ ECG

⤢ Echocardiogram—TOE > TTE

⤢ CT

⤢ MRI

Surgical management

⤢ Subxiphoid pericardial window

⤢ Thoracotomy

⤢ Video assisted thoracoscopic surgery (VATS)

9.3 Cardiac tamponade

Acute accumulation of pericardial fluid can result in tamponade.

Clinical features

⤢ ↓ Blood pressure (BP), ↑ jugular venous pressure (JVP), muffled heart sounds (Beck's triad)

⤢ Pulsus paradoxus

⤢ Tachycardia and dysrhythmias

⤢ ↓ Urine output

⤢ Widening of mediastinum on CXR

Diagnosis

⤢ Clinical examination

⤢ TTE/TOE

Management

⤢ Pericardiocentesis

⤢ Emergency thoracotomy

9.4 Lung cancer

Commonest cause of death from cancer in the UK.

Risk factors

⤢ Cigarette smoking

⤢ Radon exposure

⤢ Asbestos, aromatic hydrocarbons, arsenic

⤢ Male > female

⤢ Family history

Classification

Non-small-cell carcinoma

Squamous cell carcinoma

- 20–30% of all lung cancers
- Commonest histological type in Europe
- Arises in large airways
- Slow growing, metastasises late

Adenocarcinoma

- 30–50% of lung cancers
- Found peripherally
- Moderate growth, early metastases

Large-cell undifferentiated

- 15% of all lung cancers
- Peripheral > central
- Clear and giant cell subtypes

Small-cell carcinoma

- 20% of lung cancers
- Aggressive and not usually amenable to resection
- Pure small-cell, mixed small-cell, and large-cell subtypes

Clinical features

Proximal tumours may present with:

- Haemoptysis
- Dyspnoea
- Cough
- Wheezing
- Stridor
- Hoarseness
- Horner's syndrome
- Superior vena cava (SVC) obstruction
- Pleural effusion
- Pancoast's syndrome

Peripheral tumours are often asymptomatic, or may present with signs of chest wall invasion:

- Pleuritic pain
- Pleural effusion

Investigations

- CXR
- CT thorax
- Positron emission spectrometry (PET) scan
- Bronchoscopy
- Thoracoscopy

- ⤢ Percutaneous fine needle aspiration (FNA)/biopsy
- ⤢ Bone scan, CT abdomen/pelvis, CT head, if suspect metastases
- ⤢ Lung function tests, to determine whether proposed resection is feasible with regard to residual lung function

Treatment

Options depend on TNM staging, histopathology, and comorbidities.

Small-cell lung cancer (SCLC) responds to chemotherapy and radiotherapy. Routine resection is not recommended and should only be considered if early stage SCLC.

- ⤢ Surgical resection:
  - Nodulectomy
  - Lobectomy
  - Pneumonectomy
- ⤢ Chemotherapy
- ⤢ Radiotherapy
- ⤢ Palliative:
  - Pleurodesis
  - Chemotherapy
  - Radiotherapy

9.5 Pleural effusion

A pleural effusion is an abnormal amount of fluid within the pleural space.

Classification

Transudate (<30 g/L protein) or **exudate** (>30 g/L protein).

Light's criteria for pleural effusions:

- ⤢ Pleural fluid protein:serum protein ratio >0.5
- ⤢ Pleural fluid lactate dehydrogenase (LDH):serum LDH ratio >0.6
- ⤢ Pleural fluid LDH >200 U/L

Exudate effusions will meet at least one of the above criteria; transudate effusions should not meet any.

Causes of transudates

- ⤢ Liver cirrhosis
- ⤢ Nephritic syndrome
- ⤢ Glomerulonephritis
- ⤢ Congestive cardiac failure
- ⤢ Myxoedema
- ⤢ Sarcoidosis
- ⤢ Pulmonary emboli

Causes of exudates

- ⤢ Neoplasm—primary lung, metastatic
- ⤢ Infections—viral, bacterial, fungal, parasitic, tuberculous
- ⤢ Chylothorax
- ⤢ Haemothorax

⤢ Pulmonary emboli

⤢ Rheumatoid disease, sarcoid

Clinical features

⤢ Cough, chest pain, dyspnoea

On examination:

⤢ Decreased chest expansion

⤢ Decreased breath sounds on auscultation

⤢ Stony dullness on percussion

Investigations

⤢ CXR

⤢ USS—marking of optimal site for drainage

⤢ CT—identify underlying disease

⤢ Aspiration of pleural fluid:

- Cytology
- Protein, albumin, LDH, glucose, amylase
- Culture and sensitivity
- Gram stain
- Cell count

Treatment

⤢ Always treat underlying cause

⤢ Conservative management possible if patient asymptomatic

⤢ Chest drain insertion

⤢ If malignant cause consider pleurodesis

⤢ Thoracoscopy/thoracotomy

Chapter 10 Upper gastrointestinal pathology and physiology

10.1 Barrett's oesophagus

Barrett's oesophagus is an intestinal **metaplasia** of the oesophageal lining. The normal squamous epithelium is replaced by a gastric-type columnar epithelium.

The **squamocolumnar junction must lie >3 cm above the gastro-oesophageal junction** in order to be described as Barrett's oesophagus.

Associated with gastro-oesophageal reflux, 1 in 10 of whom will develop Barrett's oesophagus.

Dysplastic changes may eventually lead to development of adenocarcinoma. 1 in 10 with Barrett's will develop adenocarcinoma. Regular endoscopic surveillance is therefore required.

10.2 Oesophageal cancer

Types

- Adenocarcinoma (usually lower half)
- Squamous cell carcinoma (can occur anywhere)
- Lipoma/gastrointestinal stromal tumours (rare)

Risk factors

- Age (>60 years old)
- Smoking
- Alcohol
- Diet
- Gastro-oesophageal reflux disease (GORD)

Clinical features

- Dysphagia
- Weight loss
- Chest pain
- Haematemesis
- Local spread—recurrent laryngeal nerve palsy, cough, haemoptysis
- Secondary deposits—cervical lymphadenopathy, hepatomegaly, jaundice

Complications

- Obstruction
- Haemorrhage
- Fistula formation
- Lung empyema/abscesses

Investigations

- Oesophagoscopy and biopsy
- Barium swallow/meal
- CT/EUS/PET for staging

Treatment

Curative intent

- Surgical resection (oesophagectomy)
- ± Neoadjuvant chemotherapy/radiotherapy

Palliative intent

⌕ Endoscopically inserted stent

⌕ Chemotherapy/radiotherapy

Oesophageal cancer has a poor prognosis.

10.3 Oesophageal achalasia

Caused by dysfunction of the oesophageal myenteric plexus.

Lower oesophageal sphincter has high tone and is unable to relax, therefore solids and liquids cannot pass through into stomach effectively.

Peak incidence in middle-aged men and women.

Symptoms

⌕ Dysphagia

⌕ Regurgitation of undigested food

⌕ Chest pain

Investigations

⌕ Barium swallow

⌕ Oesophagogastroscopy with biopsies

⌕ Oesophageal manometry

Treatment

⌕ Medical:

- Anticholinergics, calcium channel antagonists, nitrates

⌕ Surgical:

- Heller's myotomy—laparoscopic/open
- Endoscopic pneumatic dilatation
- Endoscopic guided botulinum toxin injection

10.4 Gastro-oesophageal reflux disease

Gastric contents reflux into the oesophagus due to a weakness in the lower oesophageal sphincter or increased intra-abdominal pressure.

Risk factors

⌕ Obesity

⌕ Diet

⌕ Alcohol

⌕ Smoking

⌕ Pregnancy

Clinical features

⌕ Heartburn/indigestion

⌕ Belching/water brash

⌕ Chronic cough

⌕ Epigastric discomfort

Complications

- ↗ Barrett's oesophagus
- ↗ Oesophagitis
- ↗ Oesophageal stricture
- ↗ Dysphagia
- ↗ Peptic ulcer

Investigations

- ↗ Test for *Helicobacter pylori*
- ↗ Oesophagogastroduodenoscopy and biopsy
- ↗ Barium swallow
- ↗ Oesophageal manometry
- ↗ 24-hour oesophageal pH monitoring

Treatment

- ↗ Lifestyle modification:
  - Improve diet
  - Avoid alcohol
  - Stop smoking
  - Lose weight
  - Avoid large meals before going to sleep
- ↗ Antacids
- ↗ H2 antagonists:
  - Ranitidine
- ↗ Proton pump inhibitors (PPI):
  - Omeprazole, lanzoprazole
- ↗ If failed medical therapy:
  - Nissen fundoplication

10.5 Peptic ulcer disease

Erosion is a breach in the epithelial surface layer.

Ulceration is a breach into the submucosal layers.

Peptic ulceration can occur within the oesophagus, stomach, and first part of the duodenum.

Classification

Gastric ulceration	Associated with *H. pylori* in 45% of cases, high alcohol intake, and nonsteroidal medications
Duodenal ulceration	Associated with *H. pylori* in 85% of cases, smoking, and nonsteroidal medication

Risk factors

- ↗ *H. pylori*
- ↗ *Nonsteroidal anti-inflammatory drugs (NSAIDs)*
- ↗ GORD
- ↗ Smoking and alcohol

⌐ Family history

⌐ Zollinger–Ellison syndrome

Clinical features

⌐ Epigastric pain

⌐ Pain exacerbated by food with gastric ulceration/relieved by food in duodenal ulceration

⌐ Anorexia

⌐ Weight loss

⌐ Haematemesis/melaena

Investigations

⌐ Full blood count (FBC)

⌐ Urease test (via breath test or biopsy)

⌐ Serum IgG antibodies

⌐ Oesophagogastroduodenoscopy

⌐ Barium meal

Treatment

If confirmed *H. pylori:*

⌐ Triple eradication therapy with omeprazole, amoxicillin, metronidazole or omeprazole, clarithromycin, metronidazole

⌐ Long-term PPI

⌐ Lifestyle modification

Surgical options:

⌐ Vagotomy

⌐ Surgical resection (e.g. partial gastrectomy or total gastrectomy)

Complications

⌐ Acute upper gastrointestinal bleeding

⌐ Iron deficiency anaemia

⌐ Perforation

⌐ Gastric outlet obstruction

⌐ Carcinoma

10.6 Gastric cancer

Types

⌐ Adenocarcinoma

⌐ Neuroendocrine (carcinoid)

⌐ Leiomyoma

⌐ Gastrointestinal stromal tumour

⌐ Lymphomas

⌐ More commonly found in the antrum > body > fundus

Risk factors

- Smoking
- *H. pylori*
- Family history
- Gastric ulcer
- Diet high in salt/smoked foods

Symptoms and signs

- Dyspepsia
- Abdominal pain
- Weight loss and anorexia
- Nausea/vomiting
- Haematemesis/melaena
- Anaemia
- Possible dysphagia
- Palpable epigastric mass/supraclavicular lymphadenopathy (Troisier's sign)

Metastases

- Directly to adjacent structures
- Via lymphatic system, e.g. Virchow's node
- Blood-borne: liver, lungs

Complications

- Perforation
- Haemorrhage
- Gastric outlet obstruction

Investigations

- Oesophagogastroduodenoscopy and biopsies
- CT thorax/abdomen/pelvis
- Endoscopic ultrasonography (EUS)
- Laparoscopic staging

Treatment

Curative intent

- Total gastrectomy
- Subtotal gastrectomy

Palliative intent

- Endoscopic stent insertion for obstructive symptoms
- Gastrojejunostomy
- Endoluminal laser therapy
- Chemotherapy
- Radiotherapy

Chapter 11 Pancreatic pathology and physiology

11.1 Overview

The pancreas is an organ with exocrine and endocrine functions.

Exocrine secretions produced by acinar cells:

- Amylase
- Lipase
- Proteases

Endocrine secretions produced by Islets of Langerhans:

- Insulin (beta cells)
- Glucagon (alpha cells)
- Somatostatin (delta cells)
- Pancreatic polypeptide (PP cells)

11.2 Acute pancreatitis

The average mortality is 10–20%.

Aetiology

- Gallstones (60%)
- Alcohol (30%)
- Trauma (blunt, penetrating, iatrogenic, post ERCP)
- Pancreatic duct obstruction
- Hypercalcaemia
- Hypertryglyceraldaemia
- Drugs, e.g. steroids, diuretics, azathioprine
- Postoperative (bypass surgery)
- Viral infections (mumps, coxsackie B virus)

Clinical features

- Severe, sudden-onset epigastric pain radiating to the back
- Nausea and vomiting
- May have symptoms of obstructive jaundice

On examination:

- Tender epigastrium on palpation (may also show signs of peritonism)

If severe episode:

- Tachycardia
- Hypotension
- Oliguria
- Hypoxia
- Pyrexia

Intradermal staining by extravasated blood in flank (**Grey Turner's sign**) or at umbilicus (**Cullen's sign**) indicates retroperitoneal haemorrhage

Investigations

- Serum amylase: 3–4 times normal value
- Serum lipase: elevated for longer time compared to amylase

↗ FBC, U&Es, LFTs, Ca^{2+}, Mg^{2+}, Glucose, LDH, CRP, clotting profile

↗ Arterial blood gas

↗ CXR/AXR

↗ Rule out perforation from peptic ulcer

↗ USS abdomen may show pancreatic oedema, pancreatic mass, dilated biliary ducts, gallstones, pseudocyst

↗ CT abdomen with contrast
- As above
- Will also show evidence of necrosis/peripancreatic collections/calcification

↗ MRCP/ERCP

Remember: amylase levels can fall over 3–4 days so may not be significantly raised after an acute episode or in chronic pancreatitis.

Severity scores

Modified Glasgow score

The presence of each of the following factors scores 1 point:

↗ Age >55

↗ WBC >15 × 10^9/L

↗ Glucose >10 mmol/L

↗ Albumin <32 g/L

↗ Urea >16 mmol/L

↗ Pao_2 <8 kPa

↗ Uncorrected calcium <2 mmol/L

↗ ALT >100 IU/L

↗ LDH >600 IU/L

A score of ≥3 indicates a severe episode of pancreatitis and should prompt you to seek critical care input.

Ranson score

At admission and at 48 hours.

APACHE II

Acute physiology and chronic health evaluation score.

Treatment

↗ IV fluids

↗ Correct electrolyte imbalances

↗ Analgesia

↗ Nil by mouth or clear fluids only

↗ Nasogastric tube if vomiting profusely

↗ Urinary catheter—hourly urine output monitoring

↗ IV antibiotics—only if septic with evidence of infected collection/necrosis

↗ Insulin sliding scale-if blood sugars erratic

↗ Consider early nasojejunal feeding

↗ May require critical care support

Complications

Early

↗ Pancreatic abscess/ necrosis

↗ Sepsis

↗ Metabolic

↗ Hyperglycaemia

↗ Hypocalcaemia

↗ Ileus

↗ Acute respiratory distress syndrome (ARDS)/pleural effusions

↗ Acute renal failure

↗ Multi organ dysfunction

↗ Haemorrhage—Released pancreatic enzymes can damage blood vessels supplying the pancreas

Late

↗ Pseudocyst

↗ Enzyme-rich fluid collections arising in the lesser sac, surrounded by granulation tissue

↗ Gastric outlet obstruction

↗ Pancreatic fistula

↗ Chronic pancreatitis

> Pseudocysts <6 cm tend to self-resolve. Indications to drain them are if they become infected or very large causing obstructive symptoms. It is usually done either percutaneously or endoscopically.

11.3 Chronic pancreatitis

Chronic inflammation of the pancreas and subsequent fibrosis leads to irreversible structural changes and calcification.

Exocrine function tends to be compromised before endocrine function.

Aetiology

↗ Alcohol

↗ Repeated episodes of acute pancreatitis

↗ Biliary tract pathology

↗ Hereditary

↗ Genetic (e.g. cystic fibrosis)

↗ Malnutrition

↗ Autoimmune disease

↗ Idiopathic

Clinical features

↗ Recurrent episodes of abdominal pain

↗ Weight loss

↗ Nausea

↗ May present with symptoms of jaundice or steatorrhoea

⤢ Malnourished

⤢ May have developed diabetes mellitus

Investigations

⤢ May have normal/slightly raised serum amylase or lipase

⤢ Faecal elastase

⤢ Pancreolauryl tests

⤢ Abdominal radiograph

⤢ May show pancreatic calcification

⤢ CT abdomen with contrast

⤢ MRCP/ERCP

Treatment

⤢ Analgesia

⤢ Dietary modifications

⤢ Low-fat diet

⤢ Alcohol cessation

⤢ Pancreatin supplements

⤢ Creon

⤢ May require insulin therapy

⤢ Endoscopic dilatation or stent insertion

⤢ If stones, strictures, obstruction of ducts present

Complications

⤢ Diabetes mellitus

⤢ Malabsorption

⤢ Chronic abdominal pain

⤢ Bile duct obstruction

⤢ Pseudocyst

⤢ Duodenal obstruction

11.4 Pancreatic cancer

⤢ Poor prognosis

⤢ Patients tend to present late with metastases already present

Risk factors

⤢ Smoking

⤢ Male > female

⤢ ↑ Age with peak 60–70 years

⤢ High-fat diet

⤢ Diabetes mellitus

⤢ Alcohol excess

⤢ Chronic pancreatitis

Pathology

- 90% ductal adenocarcinoma
- 7% mucinous cystic neoplasms
- Mucinous cystadenoma/cystadenocarcinoma
- Serous cystadenoma
- Papillary cystic tumour
- 3% islet cell tumours

Location of ductal adenocarcinoma of the pancreas tends to be head > body > tail.

Clinical features

Weight loss is a common presenting symptom in pancreatic cancer.

Head of pancreas

- Obstructive jaundice due to compression/invasion of common bile duct
- May have abdominal pain

Body/tail of pancreas

- Epigastric pain radiating to the back
- Weight loss
- Steatorrhoea
- May have jaundice

Jaundice is more common in cancer of the head of the pancreas rather than the body/tail.

Other features

- Anorexia, nausea and vomiting, pruritus
- Hepatomegaly due to metastases
- Pancreatitis
- Thrombophlebitis migrans
- **Trousseau's** sign
- Splenic vein thrombosis

Investigations

- Blood tests
- FBC, U&Es, LFTs, glucose
- Tumour markers—CA 19-9
- Abdominal ultrasound
- Pancreatic mass, duct obstruction
- EUS
- Endoscopic ultrasound
- CT thorax/abdomen/pelvis with contrast

Diagnosis and staging

- Fine needle aspiration cytology (FNAC)
- Positron emission tomography (PET)
- Differentiation of neoplastic/non-neoplastic tumours
- Endoscopic retrograde cholangiopancreatography (ERCP)
- Histology and cytology
- Laparoscopy

Rule out spread before resection.

Treatment

Palliative

- Endoscopic stent insertion
- Gastrojejunostomy for duodenal obstruction
- Coeliac plexus nerve block for pain
- Radiotherapy for pain
- Chemotherapy

Curative resection

- If cancer of the pancreatic head/near the ampulla: Whipple's procedure
- If cancer of the pancreatic body/tail: distal pancretectomy

Chapter 12 **Hepatobiliary pathology**

12.1 Jaundice

Jaundice is the yellow discoloration of the skin and sclerae due to abnormally high levels of serum bilirubin (>40 mmol). Examination findings and treatment options will depend on the underlying cause of jaundice. Causes of jaundice are divided according to whether they are pre hepatic, posthepatic, or hepatic. Bilirubin is always conjugated in prehepatic jaundice, and unconjugated in posthepatic jaundice; in hepatic jaundice it can be either.

Prehepatic (haemolytic)

↗ Congenital abnormalities of red cell structure or content (e.g. sickle cell disease, hereditary spherocytosis)

↗ Autoimmune haemolytic anaemia

↗ Drug toxicity

↗ Transfusion reactions

> Always consider hepatitis in young jaundiced patients. Think about: blood transfusions, IV drug abuse, tattoos, recent foreign travel, and sexual history.

Hepatic (hepatocellular)

↗ Unconjugated:
  • Gilbert's syndrome
  • Crigler–Najar syndrome

↗ Conjugated:
  • Infections
  • Viral—hepatitis A/B/C, Epstein–Barr virus (EBV), cytomegalovirus (CMV)
  • Bacterial—liver abscesses, leptospirosis
  • Parasitic—amoebic
  • Drugs—paracetamol overdose, antipsychotics, antibiotics
  • Noninfective hepatitis, e.g. chronic active, secondary to alcohol

Posthepatic (obstructive)

↗ Intraluminal abnormalities of the bile ducts

↗ Gallstones

↗ Mural abnormalities

↗ Cholangiocarcinoma

↗ Congenital atresia

↗ Sclerosing cholangitis

↗ Biliary cirrhosis (primary and secondary)

↗ Extrinsic compression of bile ducts:
  • Pancreatitis
  • Pancreatic tumours
  • Lymphadenopathy at the porta hepatis

> Raised AST/ALT > alkaline phosphatase in hepatitis. The opposite is true in posthepatic obstruction.

Investigations

- ↗ FBC (abnormal blood film), liver function tests (deranged), clotting (↑ prothrombin time), conjugated vs unconjugated bilirubin
- ↗ In cholestasis ↑PT due to impaired vitamin K absorption
- ↗ Urinalysis
- ↗ Hepatitis screen
- ↗ USS abdomen
- ↗ MRCP
- ↗ ERCP—diagnostic and therapeutic options available
- ↗ Percutaneous transhepatic cholangiogram (PTC)
- ↗ Liver biopsy

12.2 Portal hypertension

Normal portal vein pressure is 5–10 mmHg. Portal hypertension develops when portal vein pressure is >12 mmHg.

Causes

Prehepatic

- ↗ Congenital portal vein atresia
- ↗ Portal vein thrombosis
- ↗ Occlusion by tumour or inflammation (pancreatitis)

Hepatic

- ↗ Cirrhosis
- ↗ Hepatitis
- ↗ Parasitic diseases
- ↗ Schistosomiasis

Posthepatic

- ↗ Budd–Chiari syndrome (hepatic vein thrombosis)
- ↗ Blockage of hepatic veins by tumour invasion

Pathological features

- ↗ Development of collateral portosystemic anastomoses (varices)
- ↗ Ascites
- ↗ Splenomegaly
- ↗ Hepatic failure

Investigations

- ↗ FBC, U&E, LFT's and clotting profile
- ↗ Screen for causes of cirrhosis
- ↗ Liver biopsy
- ↗ CT/USS to assess liver morphology
- ↗ Gastroscopy (assess and stop variceal bleeding)

12.3 Ascites

Defined as 'accumulation of free fluid within the peritoneal cavity'.

Combined effects of high portal pressures, low serum albumin, and sodium/water retention.

Causes

Transudate

⬈ Cirrhosis

⬈ Renal disease causing hypoalbuminaemia

⬈ Right-sided heart failure

⬈ Meig's syndrome

Exudate

⬈ Neoplasm

⬈ Infection/tuberculosis

⬈ Budd–Chiari syndrome

⬈ Pancreatitis

Clinical features

⬈ Stigmata of chronic liver disease/portal hypertension:

  • Spider naevi, caput medusae, jaundice

⬈ Large, distended abdomen:

  • Shifting dullness

  • Fluid thrill

⬈ Peripheral oedema

Investigations

⬈ Ascitic tap

⬈ White cell count (WCC)

⬈ Look for spontaneous bacterial peritonitis (SBP)

⬈ Culture and Gram stain

⬈ Protein

⬈ Amylase

⬈ Cytology

Treatment

⬈ Treat underlying cause

⬈ Paracentesis—may require albumin transfusion if large amounts of ascites drained

⬈ Fluid and sodium restriction

⬈ Diuretics:

  • Spironolactone

  • Furosemide

Child–Pugh score

⬈ Used to determine prognosis of chronic liver disease

⬈ Helps determine suitability and risk for surgery on a patient with chronic liver disease

↗ Takes into account the patient's:

- Bilirubin
- Albumin
- Prothrombin time
- Presence of ascites
- Presence of encephalopathy

↗ Grades the patient as A, B, or C depending on the levels and presence of these factors

> A favourite question format is 'What is the significance of X to the surgeon?' In this instance, the significance of ascites, i.e. the risk of surgery in hepatic-impaired patients.

12.4 Gallstones

Gallbladder

↗ Stores bile

↗ Stimulated by release of cholecystokinin to contract and release bile to aid in fat digestion/absorption

Bile

↗ Mainly composed of cholesterol, bile salts, pigments, and water

↗ Bile salts are reabsorbed in the terminal ileum (enterohepatic circulation)

Nature and formation of gallstones

↗ Affect approximately 20% of the population

↗ 80% are mixed (i.e. cholesterol/calcium)

↗ 12% are pigment stones containing bilirubin salts

↗ 8% are composed primarily of cholesterol

↗ Formation is dependent on:

- An increase in cholesterol relative to bile salts
- A nidus provided for the stones to form (e.g. bacteria)

Risk factors

> **The 5 Fs**
>
> Not the most politically correct memory aid, but a useful one to characterize the more common features of patients most likely to suffer from gallstones.
>
> ↗ Fat
>
> ↗ Female
>
> ↗ Forty
>
> ↗ Fertile
>
> ↗ Family history
>
> ↗ Others: rapid weight loss, pregnancy, diabetes, oral contraceptive pill

Clinical features

Gallstones are usually diagnosed when a patient presents with complications.

↗ Most will be asymptomatic

↗ May describe bloating or abdominal discomfort, dyspepsia, flatulence after high-fat meals

↗ May describe previous episodes of pale stools and dark urine (symptoms of obstructive jaundice)

Complications

Within the gallbladder

↗ Biliary colic

↗ Acute cholecystitis

↗ Empyema of the gallbladder

↗ Acalculous cholecystitis

↗ Mirrizi's syndrome (compression of common bile duct by a stone in the gallbladder)

↗ Mucocoele

↗ Carcinoma (0.5%)

Outside the gallbladder

↗ Pancreatitis

↗ Biliary stricture

↗ Obstructive jaundice

↗ Ascending cholangitis

↗ Gallstone ileus (this can occur when gallstone erodes into adjacent small bowel (cholecystoenteric fistula)

12.5 Biliary colic and cholecystitis

Biliary colic

↗ Occurs when a gallstone is causing irritation to the gallbladder or passing down the biliary ducts e.g. cystic duct

↗ Patient describes RUQ pain, which may last anything from 1–2 hours to 1–2 days

↗ Usually associated nausea

Clinical features

↗ Soft abdomen

↗ Mild tenderness in RUQ

↗ No signs of peritonism

↗ Afebrile

Investigations

↗ Blood tests: FBC, U&Es, CRP, LFTs, amylase

↗ Inflammatory markers should be normal

↗ LFTs usually normal but may show slight transient rise

↗ AXR—Only detects 10% of stones

↗ USS abdomen

Could be done as urgent outpatient if symptoms resolve.

Treatment

- Analgesia
- Dietary advice—low-fat diet

If symptomatic from confirmed gallstones, then should be referred to a surgeon for discussion of surgical removal of gallbladder.

Acute cholecystitis

- Infection and inflammation of the gallbladder

Clinical features

- Severe constant RUQ pain
- Fever
- Nausea and vomiting
- Pyrexia
- Tachycardia
- Tender RUQ
- Murphy's sign (indicates localized peritonism)
  - During inspiration, apply pressure over the gallbladder: patient 'catches their breath' due to the pain
- May have generalized peritonitis if perforated gallbladder
- May have signs of small-bowel obstruction if gallstone ileus (rare)

Courvoisiers' law

A palpable nontender gallbladder in the presence of jaundice is unlikely to be due to gallstones. Most often, it indicates carcinoma of the head of the pancreas.

Investigations

- Bloods: FBC, U&Es, LFTs, amylase, clotting
- CXR/AXR to rule out perforation
- USS abdomen
- May also require MRCP/ERCP if ultrasound or LFTs suggest obstructed ducts

Treatment

- IV fluids
- IV antibiotics
- Analgesia
- May require urinary catheter if septic/unwell
- Laparoscopic cholecystectomy either:
  - On acute admission <72 hours
  - 6 weeks after acute episode has settled

If obstructive LFTs or suspect intraductal stone: may require intraoperative cholangiogram or ERCP

Complications

- Gallbladder perforation/necrosis
- Gallbladder empyema
- Intra-abdominal abscess formation

Other forms of cholecystitis

Acalculous cholecystitis

↗ Usually occurs in patients who are critically ill, recent trauma, burns, major surgery

↗ Higher mortality due to increased risk of perforation/necrosis

Emphysematous cholecystitis

↗ Caused by gas-forming organisms, e.g. clostridium

↗ Poorer prognosis—high risk of perforation

↗ More common in elderly/immunocompromised patients

↗ Air seen within gallbladder wall on AXR

Ascending cholangitis

Infection and inflammation of the biliary ducts secondary to duct obstruction

Commonest cause is gallstones

Charcot's triad: fever/rigors, pain, jaundice

Management

↗ IV fluids

↗ Nil by mouth

↗ IV antibiotics

↗ Urinary catheter

↗ Early critical care input if signs of sepsis

↗ Urgent ERCP

↗ Percutaneous transhepatic cholangiogram (PTC)

12.6 Gallbladder and biliary carcinoma

Classification

Gallbladder carcinoma

↗ Most common histology:

- 90% adenocarcinoma
- 10% squamous cell

↗ Poor prognosis

Cholangiocarcinoma

↗ Carcinoma of the bile ducts

↗ Similar histology to gallbladder carcinoma

Risk factors

Gallbladder cancer

↗ Females > males

↗ Age (>60)

↗ History of gallstones

Cholangiocarcinoma

↗ History of gallstones

↗ Primary sclerosing cholangitis

↗ Ulcerative colitis

Clinical features

↗ Weight loss

↗ Jaundice, pruritus

↗ Abdominal pain

↗ Ascites

Treatment options

Surgical options are usually limited by the time patients are symptomatic, as carcinoma has already spread/metastasized.

↗ Surgical (potentially curative):

- Resection of tumour

↗ Palliative:

- Endoscopic or percutaneous stent insertion
- Radiotherapy

Chapter 13 Large bowel pathology

13.1 Appendicitis

Appendicitis is the commonest surgical emergency in developed countries. Peak age of incidence is in early teens/twenties, but it can occur in any age group.

Causes

Luminal obstruction secondary to:

- Faecoliths
- Lymphoid hyperplasia
  - Secondary to infection
- Appendix/caecal pole tumours

> **Remember:** clinical signs of appendicitis in elderly people should always raise your suspicion of carcinoma.

Clinical features

- Malaise, anorexia, and low-grade fever
- Diarrhoea and vomiting
- Abdominal pain, initially central > right iliac fossa (RIF)
- Tender/peritonitic over McBurney's point
  - 1/3 of the way along a line joining the anterior superior iliac spine and the umbilicus
- Rovsing's sign
  - Palpation of the left iliac fossa (LIF) results in pain in the RIF
- You may find palpable mass in the RIF
- Digital rectal examination (DRE):
  - May have right-sided tenderness on DRE
  - Cervical excitation may indicate pelvic inflammatory disease (PID)

> There are many differential diagnoses for young women with RIF pain; it is therefore important to be aware of common gynaecological pathologies, e.g. ectopic pregnancy, PID, Mittelschmerz, endometriosis, ovarian cysts.

Complications

- Perforation
- Appendiceal mass
- Abscess formation

Investigations

- FBC, U&Es, CRP
  - Inflammatory markers tend to be mildly raised
- Urinalysis and βHCG
  - Exclude urinary tract infection (UTI), ectopic pregnancy
- USS abdomen/pelvis
  - Can be useful to exclude pelvic pathology in women
  - May show an appendiceal mass or signs of appendiceal inflammation/oedema

⤢ CT abdomen
  • Usually used if palpable mass or carcinoma suspected
⤢ Diagnostic laparoscopy
  • If clinical diagnosis unclear or symptoms fail to improve
  • Allows direct vision of the ovaries, uterus and fallopian tubes to rule out pelvic pathology

Treatment

⤢ IV fluids and keep nil by mouth
⤢ IV antibiotics—if septic or signs of peritonism
⤢ Laparoscopic or open appendicectomy
⤢ An appendiceal abscess or inflammatory mass may be treated with IV antibiotics ± percutaneous drain insertion

If above management is successful   An interval appendicectomy can be performed in 8 weeks' time

If unsuccessful   Patient will require urgent appendicectomy

Meckel's diverticulum

Diverticulum within the ileum that contains gastric/pancreatic tissue.

⤢ Usually asymptomatic
⤢ Can sometimes present with symptoms similar to acute appendicitis

If an inflamed Meckel's diverticulum is found at surgery, small-bowel resection of the affected part is performed.

> **Features of Meckel's diverticulum**
> ⤢ 2% of population
> ⤢ 2 feet (60 cm) from ileocaecal valve
> ⤢ 2:1 male to female
> ⤢ 2 inches (5 cm) long

13.2 Diverticular disease

A diverticulum is defined as 'an abnormal outpouching of a hollow viscus into the surrounding tissues'.

A true diverticulum contains all layers of the wall of the viscus (false contains only some of the layers).

Pathology

Hypertrophy of the muscles of the sigmoid colon produces high intraluminal pressures, resulting in herniation of mucosa at site of weakness (entry point of vessels supplying the bowel wall).

⤢ **Diverticulosis** is the presence of diverticuli
  • Diverticulosis is often, but not exclusively, found in the sigmoid colon
⤢ **Diverticulitis** results from inflammation/infection of the diverticuli

Causes

⤢ Associated with low-fibre diets
⤢ More common in Western countries
⤢ More common in those >50 years old

Clinical features

Diverticulosis

⬈ Mild abdominal cramping
  - Self-limiting
⬈ Constipation
  - Stools usually 'hard pellets'
⬈ Diarrhoea

Diverticulitis

⬈ Abdominal pain—usually in LIF
⬈ Diarrhoea ± PR bleeding
⬈ Nausea ± vomiting
⬈ Malaise, decreased appetite
⬈ Fever
⬈ Tachycardia
⬈ Pyrexia
⬈ Tender on palpation of LIF:
  - May have localized peritonism
  - May have generalized peritonitis
  - May have palpable mass in LIF

Complications

⬈ Diverticular abscess
⬈ Fistula formation
⬈ Peritonitis secondary to perforation (may be localized or generalized)
⬈ Haemorrhage as a result of erosion of a vessel within the bowel wall
⬈ Obstruction

Investigations

⬈ Blood tests (FBC, U&Es, CRP):
  - Inflammatory markers raised in diverticulitis
⬈ Radiographs erect chest and abdomen
⬈ Double contrast barium enema
⬈ Flexible sigmoidoscopy/colonoscopy:
  - Becoming the preferred investigation for diagnosing diverticulosis (rather than barium enema)
⬈ CT abdomen and pelvis:
  - Commonly used in the acute setting to look for evidence of diverticulitis or diverticular abscess

Treatment

Diverticulitis is usually treated conservatively with:

⬈ IV fluids
⬈ IV antibiotics
⬈ Free fluids

Diverticulitis with perforation/abscess formation/obstruction requires IV antibiotics and fluids as well as urgent surgery; Hartmann's procedure most commonly used.

In severe diverticulosis or in a patient with frequent diverticulitis, an elective sigmoid colectomy may be performed.

Patients with diverticulosis should be advised to adopt a high-fibre diet and stay well hydrated. They may also require laxatives.

13.3 Inflammatory bowel disease

Unknown aetiology, but genetics, family history, autoimmune causes have been implicated. More common in the West.

Crohn's disease

* A chronic inflammatory, noncaseating granulomatous disease affecting any part of the alimentary tract (mouth → anus)
* Characteristic discontinuous or 'skip' lesions
* Terminal ileum most commonly affected but can affect any part of the alimentary tract.

Pathological features

* Affected bowel appears blue-grey with characteristic 'fat wrapping'
* Transmural inflammation with lymphoid aggregates
* 'Crohn's rosary'
* Mucosal crypt and fissuring ulceration
* Cobblestone appearance
* Perforation, fistulation, and abscess formation
* Fibrosis and smooth muscle hyperplasia results in stenosis
  * String sign of Kantor may be seen on barium studies, indicating spasm or stricture

Clinical features and complications

* Fever, malaise, abdominal pain
* Change in bowel habit, weight loss
* May present with perianal pathology
* Abscess formation
* Fistulas—ileocolic, ileoilieal, ileocutaneous
* Bowel obstruction
* Colon carcinoma
* Haemorrhage
* Toxic megacolon

Extraintestinal manifestations

Skin Erythema nodosum, pyoderma gangrenosum

Eyes Uveitis, iritis

Joints Arthritis, ankylosing spondylitis

Liver Sclerosing cholangitis

Investigations

- Bloods—FBC, CRP, ESR, albumin
- Flexible sigmoidoscopy/colonoscopy ± biopsy (diagnosis)
- Small-bowel enema
- Barium enema
- CT abdomen in acute episodes
  - Will detect suspected masses/abscesses
- MRI assessment of anal disease

Surgical treatment

- Not curative:
  - Often limited, conservative surgery
- Usually used to treat complications:
  - Fistula
  - Abscess
  - Stricture/obstruction
  - Toxic megacolon

Ulcerative colitis

Ulcerative colitis is an inflammatory condition affecting the colonic mucosa.

- Commonly occurs in rectum and extends proximally
- May affect ileum:
  - Backwash ileitis
- Peak incidence 20–30 years of age

Pathological features

- Hypervascular, oedematous mucosa
- Neutrophil infiltration of mucosa
- Crypt abscess formation
- Transmural inflammation
- Smooth atrophic mucosa with thinning of bowel wall

Clinical features and complications

- Diarrhoea with blood/mucus/pus
- Abdominal pain
- Weight loss
- Tenesmus
- In severe attacks:
  - Fever
  - Toxaemia
  - Bleeding
- Toxic megacolon:
  - May result in perforation
- Colon carcinoma

Extraintestinal manifestations

Skin Erythema nodosum

Eyes Uveitis, conjunctivitis

Joints Arthritis, ankylosing spondylitis

Liver Cirrhosis, sclerosing cholangitis

Investigations

⤢ Bloods:
  - FBC, CRP, ESR, albumin
  - Raised inflammatory markers
  - Anaemia

⤢ Stool cultures

⤢ AXR—oedematous colonic mucosa ('thumbprinting')

⤢ Flexible sigmoidoscopy/colonoscopy ± biopsy

⤢ Barium enema

⤢ CT abdomen in acute episodes

Surgical treatment

⤢ Curative potential

⤢ Proctocolectomy with end ileostomy

⤢ Restorative proctocolectomy with ileoanal pouch

⤢ Total colectomy with ileorectal anastomosis

⤢ In acute setting:
  - Subtotal colectomy with ileostomy

Medical management

⤢ Nutritional supplementation

⤢ Anti-inflammatories:
  - 5-ASA (aminosalicylic acid)
  - Mesalazine
  - Sulphasalazine

⤢ Immunosuppressants:
  - Steroids (prednisolone, hydrocortisone)
  - Azathioprine

⤢ Anti-TNF-α

⤢ Antibiotics

> Smoking appears to worsen symptoms in Crohn's disease and have a beneficial effect in ulcerative colitis.

13.4 Colorectal cancer

Colorectal carcinoma is the second most common cause of deaths in males after lung cancer, and the third highest in women after breast and lung cancer.

The most common histology is adenocarcinoma.

⤢ 45% occur in the rectum

⤢ 25% occur in the sigmoid colon

⤢ 20% occur in the caecum

⤢ 10% occur in the ascending > transverse > splenic flexure > descending colon

⤢ 3% of cases will have synchronous lesions

Aetiology and risk factors

⤢ 70–80% arise as a result of the polyp → cancer sequence from sporadic colonic adenomas

⤢ Familial adenomatous polyposis (FAP) and hereditary nonpolyposis colonic cancer (HNPCC)

⤢ Inflammatory bowel disease

⤢ Diet

- Low fibre

- High fat

⤢ Family history

⤢ More common > 60 years of age

Adenomas

Increased risk of transformation to adenocarcinoma with:

⤢ Size (40% risk if >2 cm)

⤢ Villous > tubulovillous > tubular adenoma

In resected specimens of colon adenocarcinoma, adenomas are also commonly found in other parts of the resected bowel.

Clinical features

⤢ Altered bowel habits

⤢ Alternating constipation/diarrhoea

⤢ Bleeding *per rectum*

⤢ Anaemia

⤢ Weight loss

⤢ Abdominal pain

⤢ May have palpable mass on examination (either abdominal or rectal)

⤢ Tenesmus

⤢ May present acutely with obstruction/perforation

Complications

⤢ Bowel obstruction

⤢ Bowel perforation and subsequent peritonitis

⤢ Haemorrhage

⤢ Metastases, e.g. lung or liver

Investigations

- ↗ FBC, LFTs:
  - Iron deficiency anaemia
  - Liver metastases
- ↗ Tumour markers:
  - Carcinoembryonic antigen (CEA)
  - CA 19.9
- ↗ Rigid sigmoidoscopy
- ↗ Flexible sigmoidoscopy
- ↗ Barium enema
- ↗ Colonoscopy (histological diagnosis)
- ↗ USS abdomen (liver metastases)
- ↗ CXR (pulmonary metastases)
- ↗ CT thorax/abdomen/pelvis (staging)

Staging

Dukes A Confined to bowel wall

Dukes B Penetration beyond muscularis propria

Dukes C Any depth and positive regional lymph nodes

Dukes D Distant spread has occurred, e.g. liver metastases

5-year survival in colorectal cancer
- ↗ Dukes A—90%
- ↗ Dukes B—70%
- ↗ Dukes C—50%

Metastases

- ↗ Direct invasion through bowel wall to adjacent structures
- ↗ Via lymphatic system
- ↗ Pulmonary metastases
- ↗ Liver metastases

Treatment

Depends on tumour staging results and patient's suitability for surgical procedure.

Curative intent
- ↗ Surgical resection of tumour with either permanent stoma or potentially reversible stoma
- ↗ Surgical resection with primary anastomosis
- ↗ Chemotherapy/radiotherapy

Palliative intent
- ↗ Noncurative surgical resection of tumour
- ↗ Defunctioning stoma, e.g. in impending obstruction
- ↗ Endoscopic stent insertion, e.g. in impending obstruction
- ↗ Chemotherapy/radiotherapy

13.5 Anorectal abscesses and fistulae

Anorectal abscess

An abscess is a localized collection of pus.

Approximately 80% are idiopathic and thought to be as a result of infection in one of the anal glands.

Approximately 20% are secondary to specific causes:

- IBD (Crohn's)
- Fissure
- Trauma
- Following anorectal surgery
- Immunocompromised patients

Classification

- Subcutaneous/perianal (60%)
- Ischiorectal (30%)
- Intersphincteric (5%)
- Supralevator (2%)
- Deep postanal (1%)

Anorectal fistulae

A fistula is an abnormal connection between two epithelial lined surfaces.

Most occur as a result of anorectal abscesses.

May occur secondary to conditions such as Crohn's, TB, or carcinoma.

Classification

- Intersphincteric
- Transsphincteric
- Suprasphincteric
- Extrasphincteric

Treatment

Simple perianal or ischirectal abscesses require incision and drainage under general anaesthetic.

Anorectal fistulae will require EUA (CHECK!!!) rectum ± seton insertion.

Complex anorectal fistulae may require further assessment with endoanal ultrasound or MRI.

13.6 Haemorrhoids

Overview

The anal canal submucosa forms a series of 'cushions', commonly found at the 3, 7, and 11 o'clock positions. The cushions are made up of:

- Anorectal mucosa
- Submucosal tissue
- Submucosal blood vessels

Haemorrhoids (piles) are prolapsed anal cushions.

Classification

According to location in anal canal

Internal   Above the dentate line

External   Below the dentate line

Internal–external Mixture of above types

According to degree of prolapse

First degree Project into lumen during straining, but do not prolapse

Second degree Prolapse during defecation, then reduce into anal canal spontaneously

Third degree Prolapse during defecation, require manual reduction

Fourth degree Prolapsed and irreducible

Clinical features

- Bleeding during/after defecation (bright red) and separate from stool
- Prolapse
- Mucous discharge
- Pruritus ani
- Perianal pain and discomfort
- Thrombosed piles are tender, painful, and swollen

Investigations

- Rigid sigmoidoscopy
- Proctoscopy

Treatment

- Conservative management
  - High-fibre diet/laxatives
  - Anusol cream/suppositories
  - Ice packs
- Banding/injection sclerotherapy:
  - For first- or second-degree haemorrhoids
- Haemorrhoidectomy:
  - For third- or fourth-degree haemorrhoids

Thrombosed piles will often settle with conservative treatment and are rarely managed with a haemorrhoidectomy in the acute setting.

13.7 Anal fissure

Overview

- Mucosal tear within the anal canal
- 90% are on posterior wall
- Increased risk with constipation, pregnancy, inflammatory bowel disease, sexually transmitted infections
- May develop a sentinel pile

Treatment

⤢ Conservative
- High-fibre diet
- Keep well hydrated
- Stool softeners
- Glyceryl trinitrate (GTN) cream
- Diltiazem ointment

⤢ Botulinum injection

⤢ Lateral sphincterotomy

13.8 Stomas

A **stoma** (Greek for mouth) is an artificial union made between two conduits, or between a conduit and the outside.

Stomas are commonly found in OSCE stations, so make sure you are familiar with recognizing and describing them.

Site

In the selection of stoma site the following areas should be avoided:

⤢ Bony prominences

⤢ Umbilical region

⤢ Scars

⤢ Skin folds/creases

⤢ Waist/trouserline

Colostomies

End colostomy

The bowel is divided and the proximal end brought out as a stoma. The distal portion of the bowel may be:

⤢ Resected (abdominoperineal resection)

⤢ Closed and left within the abdomen (Hartman's procedure)

⤢ Exteriorized (mucous fistula)

Loop colostomy

A loop of colon is exteriorized, opened, and sewn to the skin. A plastic rod may be placed beneath the loop to prevent retraction.

Double-barrelled colostomy

The proximal part of the bowel is brought out as a stoma and the distal part is also brought out through the same opening in the abdominal wall as a mucous fistula.

⤢ May look very similar to a loop colostomy

Ileostomies

Ileostomies emit small-bowel content, which is rich in digestive enzymes. They are therefore spouted (protrude from skin) to avoid excoriation of the surrounding skin.

End ileostomy

May be formed following a panproctocolectomy or subtotal colectomy for ulcerative colitis.

Loop ileostomy

Can be used to relieve a distal obstruction or protect a distal anastomosis.

Urostomies

Fashioned after cystectomy; allows urine to pass from the ureters to a bag on the abdominal wall via an ileal conduit.

Complications

Early

⤢ Haemorrhage

⤢ Ischaemia

⤢ High output

⤢ Obstruction

⤢ Retraction

Late

⤢ Obstruction

⤢ Surrounding dermatitis

⤢ Prolapse

⤢ Parastomal hernia

⤢ Fistulae

⤢ Psychological

Chapter 14 Urological pathology and physiology

14.1 Prostate gland

↗ Two-thirds glandular components, one-third fibromuscular

↗ Normal weight approximately 20 g

↗ Its secretions form nearly one-third of the total volume of seminal fluid

Prostate specific antigen (PSA)

↗ A glycoprotein that is a serine protease

↗ Secreted by the prostate gland

↗ Helps sperm to travel by liquefying semen

Serum levels of PSA depend on the size of the prostate gland and the effectiveness of the barrier between prostate and serum. In prostate cancer the barrier is weakened.

Causes of raised PSA

↗ Prostatitis

↗ Benign prostatic hyperplasia (BPH)

↗ Prostate cancer

↗ UTI

↗ Recent catheterization/cystoscopy

↗ Age

> Checking a patient's PSA has serious implications and should not be done without the patient's knowledge and appropriate discussion/ counselling beforehand.

14.2 Benign prostatic hyperplasia

BPH is a nonmalignant enlargement of the prostate gland (increase in **stromal and glandular** components). It is the commonest cause of lower urinary tract symptoms in middle aged and elderly men. The aetiology is unknown.

Clinical features

↗ Frequency, urgency, nocturia, and incontinence

↗ Hesitancy, poor stream, terminal dribbling

↗ Chronic/ acute urinary retention secondary to bladder outlet obstruction (BOO)

↗ On examination:

• Diffusely enlarged smooth gland on digital rectal examination (DRE)

• Palpable bladder (if in retention)

Complications

↗ Lower urinary tract symptoms

↗ Haematuria

↗ UTI

↗ Urinary retention

↗ Overflow incontinence

↗ Postrenal failure

Investigations
- DRE
- PSA
- Urinalysis/MSU
- Serum urea/creatinine (raised in postrenal failure)
- Postvoid residual volume
  - >300 mL indicates chronic retention
- Urodynamics
  - Max flow rate of <10 mL consistent with BOO
- Cystoscopy (exclude bladder disease)
- Transrectal ultrasound guided biopsy (exclude malignancy)
- Renal USS (may show evidence of hydronephrosis due to obstruction)

Medical treatment
- α-Blockers (tamsulosin, doxazosin):
  - Target α_1-adrenergic receptors and cause relaxation of the prostatic smooth muscle
- 5α-Reductase inhibitors (finasteride, dutasteride):
  - Prevent conversion of testosterone to dihydrotestosterone
  - Help to reduce the size of the prostate

Surgical treatment
- Indications:
  - Severe symptoms or high residual volumes (>800 mL)
  - Failed medical therapy
  - Chronic retention causing renal impairment
  - Failed trial without catheter (TWOC)
- Transurethral resection of prostate (TURP):
  - Complications include bleeding, urosepsis, urethral stricture, retrograde ejaculation, impotence, and TUR syndrome
- Open prostatectomy (prostate >100 g)

> **TUR syndrome**
> This occurs due to excess absorption of irrigation fluid in TURPs and can result in hyponatraemia, hypervolaemia, and cerebral oedema. Treatment is with diuretics and fluid restriction ± critical care support.

14.3 Prostate cancer
- Most common cancer affecting males in the Western world
- Commonly affects peripheral zone of prostate gland
- Adenocarcinoma in >95%

Risk factors
- Age
- Race: African/mixed race > white/Asian

    ↗ Genetics/family history

    ↗ Diet

Clinical features

    ↗ Similar to those of BPH

    ↗ Lower urinary tract symptoms

    ↗ Haematuria

    ↗ Chronic/acute urinary retention

    ↗ Bone pain/cord compression secondary to metastatic disease

    ↗ On examination:

       ● Hard, craggy prostate

       ● May find firm nodules palpated on DRE

Investigations

    ↗ Blood tests:

       ● Serum PSA (high sensitivity, low specificity)

       ● U&E's, raised in postrenal failure

       ● LFTs, alkaline phosphatase, calcium—may be deranged if metastases present

    ↗ Transrectal USS and biopsy:

       ● Risks: bleeding, infection, systemic sepsis in 1%

    ↗ CT thorax, abdomen, and pelvis

    ↗ MRI

       ● To assess extracapsular spread

    ↗ Isotope bone scan:

       ● To look for presence of bone metastases

       ● Indicated in patients with Gleason score ≥8 or PSA >15

    ↗ Skeletal radiographs:

       ● Again, to look for metastases

> **Remember:** in prostate cancer, bone metastases are osteoblastic (↑ bone density).

Metastases

Periprostatic invasion	Urethra, bladder, seminal vesicles
Lymphatic spread	Iliac, sacral, para-aortic lymph nodes
Blood-borne spread	Pelvis, sacrum, spine, femur, lungs, liver

Staging

Gleason score (histopathological grade)

    ↗ The most common histological pattern is assigned the primary Gleason grade

    ↗ The next most common pattern is assigned a secondary Gleason grade

    ↗ Gleason grade ranges from 1 (well differentiated) to 5 (poorly differentiated)

    ↗ These are then combined to form the Gleason score (total range 2–10)

    ↗ The higher the Gleason score, the worse the prognosis

A Gleason score of 4 + 3 = 7 has a poorer prognosis than a score of 3 + 4 = 7, as more of the tissue is of a higher grade dysplasia.

TNM staging

The Tumour, Node, Metastases (TNM) staging system is commonly used for staging prostate cancer.

You should familiarize yourself with the TNM staging for both prostate cancer and bladder cancer.

Treatment options

Localized prostate cancer

↗ Radical prostatectomy—open, laparoscopic, robotic (da Vinci)
↗ External beam radiotherapy ± hormone therapy
↗ Brachytherapy ± hormone therapy
↗ Active surveillance—regular PSA/biopsies

Locally advanced prostate cancer

↗ Radical external beam radiotherapy ± hormone therapy (LHRH analogue)
↗ Androgen ablation (medical or surgical)
↗ Radical prostatectomy—if young and minimal advancement
↗ Active surveillance—if low life expectancy and minimal symptoms

Metastatic prostate cancer

↗ Medical castration—LHRH analogues
↗ Surgical castration—orchidectomy
↗ Radiotherapy—for bone pain or excessive bleeding

Spinal bone metastases may cause cord compression and require dexamethasone ± surgical decompression.

14.4 Bladder cancer

Bladder cancer is the second most common urological malignancy in the UK.

It is the fourth most common cancer in men and the eleventh most common cancer in women.

Classification

↗ Transitional cell carcinoma (TCC):
  • Accounts for > 90% of bladder cancers
  • If a TCC is found in the bladder there is an increased risk of a further urothelial tumour in the upper tract
↗ Carcinoma *in situ* (CIS):
  • Carries a high risk of progression to an invasive tumour
↗ Adenocarcinoma:
  • Less than 2% of bladder tumours
↗ Squamous cell carcinoma (SCC):
  • 1% of bladder cancers in the UK

Risk factors

- Gender—males > females
- Age—average age at diagnosis 65 years
- Ethnicity   More common in white Europeans
- Smoking:
  - The greatest risk factor for bladder cancer in the UK
- Occupational exposure:
  - Aromatic amines in the rubber, textile, dye, leather, printing, solvent, and petroleum industries
- Trauma, inflammation, infection:
  - Indwelling catheter, bladder stones, or chronic infection are all associated with a higher risk of developing SCC
  - *Schistoma haematobium* is also believed to increase the risk of SCC

> Inexplicably, the occupational risk factors of cancers seem to be a recurring favourite of the examiners!

Clinical features

- Haematuria
  - More than 80% of cases present in this way (painless, gross haematuria)
  - Usually intermittent episodes
  - May be microscopic haematuria
  - Lower urinary tract symptoms (usually found in the presence of CIS or advanced bladder cancer)
- Pain
  - Loin pain if a bladder tumour has caused an obstruction to a ureter and resulted in hydronephrosis
- Advanced symptoms
  - Lower limb swelling secondary to iliac vessel compression from a tumour or lymphatic obstruction
  - Bone pain may be an indication of metastatic disease
- On examination:
  - Usually unremarkable—clinical signs normally found in advanced disease
  - Pale conjunctivae due to anaemia—blood lost from haematuria, chronic renal failure, or bone marrow infiltration secondary to metastatic disease
  - On examining the abdomen a mass may be felt suprapubically, or also on rectal and vaginal examination
  - Check for lymphadenopathy or hepatomegaly—may indicate metastatic disease

Investigations

- Urinalysis and MSU
- Urine cytology
- Blood tests—U&Es, alkaline phosphatase, calcium, LFTs, FBC
- USS urinary tract—may show hydronephrosis or bladder filling defects
- Flexible cystoscopy—if tumour identified then may require rigid cystoscopy and transurethral resection of bladder tumour (TURBT)

⌁ CT abdomen/pelvis—for staging

⌁ MRI—better than CT for staging muscle-invasive carcinoma

⌁ Skeletal radiographs and isotope bone scan—if suspect metastases

Staging

Bladder tumours are graded using the 1973 WHO grading system. They can be classified as G1, G2, and G3 which corresponds to well, moderately and poorly differentiated tumour.

The 2002 TNM staging system is widely accepted as the primary reference to the histological staging of a bladder carcinoma.

Transitional cell carcinomas can also be broadly classified as:

⌁ Superficial (Ta, T1, CIS, N0/M0)

⌁ Muscle-invasive (T2, T3, T4, N0/N1, M0)

⌁ Advanced metastatic (Ta–T4, N2/N3, M1)

Treatment options

Superficial TCC

⌁ Rigid cystoscopy and TURBT (gold standard)

⌁ Intravesical chemotherapy:

  • Mitomycin C

⌁ Intravesical immunotherapy:

  • Bacille Calmette–Guérin

Muscle-invasive TCC

⌁ Radical cystectomy and lymph node dissection

⌁ External beam radiotherapy—if significant comorbidities/not suitable for surgery

⌁ Systemic chemotherapy:

  • The two regimens frequently used are methotrexate, vinblastine, adriamycin, cisplatin (MVAC) and gemcitabine, cisplatin (GC)

14.5 Testicular cancer

⌁ Peak incidence 20–50 years of age

⌁ 90–95% are germ cell tumours

Risk factors

⌁ Age

⌁ Ethnicity—white > Afro-Caribbean

⌁ Family history

⌁ Crypto-orchidism (risk still increased even if previously corrected)

Clinical features

⌁ Painless testicular swelling

⌁ May have secondary hydrocele

⌁ May present as unresolved epididymo-orchitis

⌁ Gynaecomastia

⌁ Symptoms from metastases—lung metastases

Classification

Primary

⬈ Germ cell tumours

- Seminoma

⬈ Nonseminomatous germ cell tumours (NSGCT)

- Embryonal carcinoma
- Teratoma
- Yolk sac tumour
- Choriocarcinoma

⬈ Non-germ-cell tumour

- Leydig cell tumour
- Sertoli cell tumour
- Gonadoblastoma

Secondary

⬈ Lymphoma

⬈ Leukaemic infiltration

⬈ Metastatic

Never perform trans-scrotal biopsy, because of the risk of seeding.

Investigations

⬈ USS testes

⬈ CT thorax, abdomen, pelvis—for staging

⬈ CXR—look for pulmonary metastases

⬈ Tumour markers (AFP, βHCG, LDH, PLAP)

⬈ Alpha-fetoprotein—may be raised in NSGCT

⬈ Beta-human chorionic gonadotropin (βHCG)—may be raised in NSGCT and about 10% of seminomas

⬈ Lactic acid dehydrogenase—indicator of tumour bulk

⬈ Placental alkaline phosphatase—may be raised in seminoma

⬈ Gamma-glutamyl transpeptidase

Remember: AFP is not raised in seminoma.

Staging

Royal Marsden Hospital Staging is a commonly used simple staging system.

I	No evidence of disease outside testes
IM	As above, but with persistently raised tumour markers
II	Infradiaphragmatic node involvement
III	Supra- and infradiaphragmatic node involvement
IV	Extralymphatic metastases

Treatment

- Radical orchidectomy
  - Always inguinal approach as scrotal approach would risk seeding and inguinal metastases
- Chemotherapy
  - Bleomycin, etoposide, cisplatin (BEP)

14.6 Hydrocele and varicocele

Hydrocele

A serous fluid collection within the tunica vaginalis.

Broadly classified as:

- Primary (idiopathic)
- Secondary (due to trauma, infection, or neoplasm)

Four common types:

- Vaginal:
  - Commonest type
  - Commonly due to primary pathology
  - Occasionally secondary to tumour, orchitis, or torsion
- Congenital:
  - Associated with a patent processus vaginalis
- Infantile:
  - The processus vaginalis is obliterated at the deep ring, resulting in a fluid collection anterior to the testes and cord
- Hydrocele of the cord:
  - Occurs when part of the processus vaginalis separates leaving a fluid collection at that site

Treatment

- If small—consider conservative management
- If large and affecting quality of life—surgical repair
- No point in aspirating as it will undoubtedly reoccur
- If secondary hydrocele—treat initial cause

Varicocele

A varicose dilatation of the pampiniform plexus/cremasteric veins.

- Often described as similar to a 'bag of worms' on palpation
- Association with decreased fertility
- 95% arising on the left side:
  - May be secondary to absent valves in the terminal left testicular vein
  - Left testicular vein enters the left renal vein at almost right angles whereas the right testicular vein enters the IVC directly at a shallower angle

Treatment

- Conservative
- Surgical varicocele repair
- Radiological embolization

In elderly patients with a varicocele a renal USS should be requested, as sometimes an underlying renal carcinoma may be the cause.

14.7 Renal calculi

Risk factors

- Diet—high-protein, oxalate-rich foods
- Dehydration
- Previous renal stones
- Metabolic abnormalities—hyperparathyroidism
- Male > female
- Crohn's disease
- Family history

Clinical features

- Sudden-onset 'loin to groin' pain
- Patients usually restless—cannot get comfortable
- Haematuria
- Fever/tachycardia
- Nausea and vomiting
- Lower urinary tract symptoms (LUTS)

Remember: loin/groin pain in elderly patients with no history of renal stones may well be caused by an underlying abdominal aortic aneurysm.

Composition

- Calcium oxalate—most stones are calcium based
- Calcium phosphate
- Mixed calcium oxalate/ phosphate
- Magnesium ammonium phosphate—struvite (associated with proteus urinary infections)
- Uric acid—urate stones are not radio-opaque
- Cystine
- Xanthine

The three most common sites in the ureter for stones to become obstructive are the **pelvi-ureteric junction**, the **level of the sacroiliac joint where ureter crosses the iliacs**, and the **vesico-ureteric junction.**

Investigations

- Urinalysis—90% will have haematuria
- Serum calcium, urate, phosphate
- FBC, U&Es, CRP
- KUB radiograph—90% of stones are radio-opaque
- Intravenous urography (IVU)

↗ Renal tract USS—to look for evidence of hydronephrosis

↗ CT KUB—fast becoming the gold standard investigation

Treatment options

> Renal stones >4 mm are unlikely to pass of their own accord.

Initial management

↗ Analgesia

- Diclofenac 100 mg PR (if renal function normal)

↗ IV fluids

↗ IV antibiotics—if febrile and raised inflammatory markers

Further management

↗ If pain not resolving or deranged renal function:

- Urgent cystoscopy and ureteric stent insertion

↗ If septic with an obstructed ureter:

- Urgent nephrostomy

↗ If pain settles and patient is well:

- Conservative management
- Consider discharging with a follow-up in Outpatients with repeat KUB radiograph
- Tamsulosin 400 µg OD can help patients to pass stones if they are small and in the distal ureter

Long-term management

↗ Extracorporeal shock wave lithotripsy

↗ Percutaneous nephrolithotomy

↗ Ureteroscopy/laser fragmentation

Chapter 15 Hernias and intestinal obstruction

15.1 Hernias

A hernia is the protrusion of a viscus through an abnormal defect or weakness in its surrounding structures.

Differential diagnoses of groin lumps

⤴ Inguinal hernia

⤴ Femoral hernia

⤴ Saphena varix

⤴ Enlarged lymph node

⤴ Psoas abscess

⤴ Femoral aneurysm

⤴ Lipoma of cord

⤴ Undescended testicle

⤴ Hydrocele of canal of Nuck

Aetiology

⤴ Increased intra-abdominal pressure:
  - Chronic cough (COPD)
  - Heavy lifting
  - Constipation
  - Pregnancy/ascites

⤴ Weakness in muscles/fascia:
  - Smoking
  - Elderly
  - Malnutrition
  - Collagen defects (AAA)

Complications

⤴ Incarceration/obstruction:
  - Hernia becomes trapped and irreducible; if contents include bowel, then may cause obstructive symptoms

⤴ Strangulation:
  - Hernia is trapped and irreducible, and blood supply to its contents has become constricted; necrosis can therefore occur

Other types of hernia

Incisional

⤴ Occurs when a weak surgical or traumatic wound allows peritoneum to protrude through

⤴ Predisposing factors:
  - Post-op haematoma
  - Wound infection
  - Poor technique (tissues sutured under tension)

Para-umbilical

⤴ Occurs through a defect in the linea alba

⤴ Usually as a result of obesity or raised intra-abdominal pressure

Epigastric
↗ Occurs in the midline through defects in the linea alba
↗ Usually halfway between the umbilicus and xiphoid process

Spigelian
↗ Occurs through the linea semilunaris

15.2 Inguinal hernia

Inguinal and femoral anatomy has been covered in other chapters. Make sure you understand and remember it, as examiners love to ask questions such as 'What are the anatomical borders of the inguinal canal?'

Overview
↗ Commonest type of groin hernia
↗ Hernia sac may contain omentum/bowel/bladder
↗ Two types: direct and indirect

Direct inguinal hernia
↗ More common in male adults
↗ Neck of sac arises lateral to inferior epigastric artery
↗ Hernia protrudes through area of Hesselbach's triangle (weakness in transversalis fascia)

Indirect inguinal hernia
↗ More common in male children
↗ Neck of sac arises medial to inferior epigastric artery
↗ Travels from deep ring to superficial ring to scrotum

Clinical features
↗ Painless or painful lump in groin
↗ May be reducible or irreducible
↗ May disappear when lying flat
↗ Vomiting/unable to pass flatus—may indicate obstruction
↗ Always examine patient standing and supine
↗ Determine if hernia arising above and medial or below and lateral to pubic tubercle
↗ Is hernia soft/hard/tender/reducible?
↗ Is there a cough impulse?

Management
↗ Conservative—if elderly and asymptomatic

Surgical repair
↗ Most common operation is Lichenstein repair with Prolene mesh
  • Can be performed under local anaesthetic/sedation if necessary
↗ Other methods:
  • Shouldice repair
  • Laparoscopic hernia repair—if recurrent hernia or bilateral hernias

Complications of surgery

- ↗ Haematoma
- ↗ Wound infection/mesh infection
- ↗ Urinary retention
- ↗ Chronic pain:
  - Can occur if ilioinguinal nerve not spared
- ↗ Reccurrence of hernia
- ↗ Testicular atrophy, ichaemic orchitis, impotence

15.3 Femoral hernia

Features

- ↗ Commoner in women
- ↗ Usually irreducible, hard lump below and lateral to pubic tubercle
- ↗ May not exhibit a cough impulse
- ↗ High risk of strangulation:
  - Three of the four walls of the femoral canal are relatively rigid, predisposing to strangulation

Management

- ↗ Surgical repair due to high risk of strangulation
- ↗ In emergency situation:
  - McEvedy's repair: easier to access bowel and perform resection if required
- ↗ In elective situation:
  - Lothiessens approach
  - Lockwood approach

15.4 Intestinal obstruction

Pathophysiology

- ↗ Proximal dilatation occurs above the obstructing lesion
- ↗ Distal bowel collapses
- ↗ Subsequent accumulation of gas and fluid and reduced reabsorption
- ↗ Dilatation of gut wall producing mucosal oedema
- ↗ Impairment of arterial and venous flow
- ↗ Ischaemia, infarction, and perforation of the bowel
- ↗ Translocation of bacteria and endotoxins

Causes

- ↗ Small-bowel obstruction (SBO):
  - Adhesions
  - Hernias
  - Malignancy
  - Crohn's
  - Gallstones

⤤ Large-bowel obstruction (LBO):

- Malignancy
- Diverticulitis/strictures
- Sigmoid/caecal volvulus
- Hernias
- Gallstones
- Acute colonic pseudo-obstruction (Ogilvie's syndrome)

Clinical features

⤤ Abdominal pain—colicky in nature

⤤ Variable degree of abdominal distension

⤤ Vomiting

- Presents earlier in SBO and later in LBO

⤤ Absolute constipation:

- Presents earlier in LBO and later in SBO

⤤ Dehydrated

⤤ Hypotension, tachycardia

⤤ Loud, tinkling active bowel sounds

⤤ May have signs of peritonism if bowel necrosis/ischaemia

Investigations

⤤ Blood tests:

- FBC, U&Es, magnesium, group and save, LFTs, CRP

⤤ Consider arterial blood gas

⤤ Abdominal radiograph:

- Small bowel identified by its valvulae coniventes which cross the entire width of the bowel
- Diameter >3 cm indicates obstruction
- Large bowel identified by its haustral pattern which does not cross the entire width of the bowel
- Diameter >6 cm indicates obstruction

⤤ CT abdomen with oral and IV contrast:

- Helps identify the transition point of the obstruction as well as the underlying cause

Laplace's law

In LBO, if the ileocaecal valve is competent, the maximum dilatation will be at the caecum so this is where the bowel is most likely to perforate.

Management

⤤ IV fluids

⤤ Keep nil by mouth

⤤ Nasogastric tube

⤤ Urinary catheter

⤤ Analgesia/antiemetic

⌐ Correct electrolyte imbalances

⌐ Conservative:

• If partial obstruction and no signs of peritonism may consider 'drip and suck' to see if obstruction resolves

⌐ Surgical:

• If unresolving or complete obstruction with signs of peritonism—urgent laparotomy and proceed

15.5 Ileus and pseudo-obstruction

Loss of peristaltic function in small or large bowel.

Small-bowel ileus

⌐ Common after abdominal surgery

⌐ Intra-abdominal collections/peritonitis

⌐ Electrolyte imbalance (especially potassium)

⌐ Drugs

Features

⌐ Similar to SBO

⌐ Vomiting

⌐ Abdominal distension

⌐ Constipation

⌐ Usually quiet bowel sounds

⌐ Abdomen should not show signs of peritonism

Management—conservative

⌐ Correct electrolyte imbalances

⌐ Nasogastric (NG) tube

⌐ IV fluids

⌐ Consider total parenteral nutrition (TPN) if prolonged ileus

Large-bowel pseudo-obstruction

Causes

⌐ Drugs—opiates, antidepressants

⌐ Electrolyte disturbances—especially potassium

⌐ Retroperitoneal haematoma

⌐ Parkinson's disease

⌐ Scleroderma

Features

⌐ Patients usually elderly with multiple comorbidities, bedridden

⌐ Constipation

⌐ Abdominal distension

⌐ Vomiting

Management

- Treat underlying cause
- Correct electrolytes
- Review medications
- NG tube
- May require decompression with flatus tube or colonoscopy
- May require enema

Chapter 16 **Vascular pathology**

16.1 Abdominal aortic aneurysm

An aneurysm is a localized dilatation of a blood vessel to more than twice the normal diameter.

True aneurysms Contain all three layers of the arterial wall

False aneurysms Secondary to trauma, injury, or infection (periarterial haematoma)

Classification

Most abdominal aortic aneurysms (AAA) are infrarenal (95%)

Other common sites for aneurysms:

⬈ Iliac

⬈ Femoral

⬈ Renal

⬈ Popliteal

Risk factors

⬈ Smoking

⬈ Hypertension

⬈ Diabetes mellitus

⬈ Hyperlipidaemia

⬈ Connective tissue disorders

Clinical features

⬈ Asymptomatic:

  ● May be discovered incidentally

⬈ Symptomatic:

  ● From compression of adjacent structures

⬈ If acute rupture:

  ● Collapse/shock

  ● Abdominal pain

  ● 70% mortality before arrival at hospital

Investigations

⬈ In a nonacute situation:

  ● AXR—look for calcification of the aneurysmal wall

  ● USS abdomen

  ● CT abdomen

  ● CT angiography

⬈ In an acute situation:

  ● Immediate surgical repair

  ● Nothing should delay patient going straight to theatre if haemodynamically unstable and AAA rupture suspected

  ● Try to cross-match patient; otherwise will need O negative blood

Treatment

⬈ Risk of rupture is related to aortic diameter—surgical repair required if >5.5 cm

↗ CT angiography will delineate the extent of the aneurysm and facilitate preoperative planning

↗ If <5.5 cm then 6-monthly USS and regular surveillance

Complications

↗ Fistula into IVC or bowel

↗ Compression of adjacent structures

↗ Renal failure

↗ Death—85% overall mortality for ruptured AAA

16.2 Aortic dissection

In aortic dissection there is a tear in the intimal lining. Blood collects in the media and the dissection can extend both proximally and distally.

↗ Can be present for up to 2 years but usually presents acutely

↗ Most common site is 2–3 cm from aortic valve

Classification

Stanford classification

Type A   Origin of dissection affects ascending aorta

Type B   Origin of dissection beyond the aortic arch

Debakey classification

Type 1   Origin in ascending aorta and involves aortic arch ± descending aorta

Type 2   Confined to the ascending aorta

Type 3   Only involves descending aorta (origin beyond left subclavian artery branch)

Risk factors

↗ Smoking

↗ Hypertension

↗ Connective tissue disorders:

↗ Marfan's syndrome, Ehlers–Danlos

↗ Trauma

↗ Post cardiac angiography/cardiac surgery

Clinical features

↗ Shortness of breath

↗ Sudden-onset 'tearing' chest pain/interscapular pain

↗ Shock/collapse

↗ Neurological symptoms, e.g. stroke

Investigations

↗ ECG

↗ CXR

↗ Widened mediastinum

↗ Transoesophageal echocardiogram

↗ Angiography

Treatment

- ↗ If Stanford type A:
  - Usually requires surgery
- ↗ If Stanford type B and stable dissection:
  - Manage medically—antihypertensives

Complications

- ↗ Haemorrhage
- ↗ Cardiac tamponade
- ↗ Death
- ↗ Ischaemic changes to upper limbs, neurological symptoms, CVA:
  - Dissection may involve branches of left braciocephalic, left common carotid, left subclavian arteries

16.3 Coarctation of the aorta

Congenital narrowing of the aorta at the level of the ligamentum areteriosum. Usually found in children/young adults.

Clinical features

- ↗ Hypertension
- ↗ Complications associated with long-term hypertension, e.g. stroke, coronary artery disease
- ↗ Clinical findings will depend on position of narrowing:
  - If after branch to left subclavian artery patient would have bilateral delay in radio-femoral pulses
  - If before left subclavian artery, patient may have radio-radio delay and right-sided radio-femoral delay

Investigations

- ↗ ECG
- ↗ CXR
  - May show rib 'notching' where parts of the ribs are reabsorbed/eroded due to increased blood flow
- ↗ Echocardiogram
- ↗ CT angiogram or MR angiogram

Treatment

- ↗ Conservative
  - Medical management of hypertension
- ↗ Surgery
- ↗ Angioplasty

16.4 Carotid artery stenosis

Commonest area for atheroma and stenosis is at the common carotid artery bifurcation.

Risk factors

- Smoking
- Hypertension
- Hyperlipidaemia

Clinical features

- Asymptomatic
- Neurological symptoms, e.g. transient ischaemic attack, paraesthesia, limb weakness, dysphasia, stroke
- Amaurosis fugax:
  - 'Curtain coming down'
  - Transient loss of vision
- Patients may have a carotid bruit on auscultation

Investigations

- USS Doppler
- MR angiogram/CT angiogram

Treatment

- Commence antiplatelet therapy
- Commence statin
- If symptomatic (recent TIA, nondisabling stroke) with 70–99% stenosis:
  - Carotid endarterectomy (CEA) may be indicated
- If asymptomatic:
  - CEA controversial in asymptomatic patients
  - If <60% stenosis—medical management
  - If 60–80% stenosis—consider regular Doppler USS to look for progression or worsening despite medical treatment
  - >80% stenosis—consider CEA

16.5 Varicose veins

Dilated, tortuous veins that commonly follow the distribution of the long and short saphenous veins. Increased venous pressure causes venous dilatation and subsequent valvular incompetence.

Risk factors

- Age
- Female > male
- Previous deep vein thrombosis (DVT)
- Obesity
- Pregnancy

Clinical features

- Usually asymptomatic but cosmetically unpleasant
- May have discomfort/heaviness in lower limbs
- Venous eczema/lipodermatosclerosis
- Itching/bleeding
- Saphena varix

Investigations

- Colour flow duplex scan

Treatment

Conservative

- Compression stockings
- Injection sclerotherapy

Surgical treatment

- Ligation of saphenous vein and perforating veins at saphenofemoral junction
- Stripping of saphenous vein above knee
- Avulsion of perforating veins below knee

16.6 Mesenteric ischaemia

A condition in which segments of intestine become ischaemic secondary to vascular insufficiency. Ischaemia may be focal or diffuse.

Acute focal ischaemia

Arises from mechanical intestinal obstruction secondary to hernias, adhesive bands or volvulus. The wall of the bowel becomes ischaemic, predisposing it to perforation.

Clinical features

- Loss of serosal lustre
- Lack of peristalsis
- Absence of mesenteric arterial pulsation
- Purple/black discoloration (not reliable)

Acute diffuse ischaemia

- Secondary to thrombosis or embolism
- Embolus can arise from a mural thrombus (post MI) or as a result of atrial fibrillation

Clinical features

- Abdominal pain:
  - Poorly localized
  - May be intermittent in chronic ischaemia
  - Usually severe in acute ischaemia
  - Postprandial
- Nausea/vomiting
- Diarrhoea
- May have generalized peritonitis, abdominal distension, perforation, shock, haemodynamic instability

Investigations

- Bloods
  - FBC, U&E's, LFT, CRP, amylase, G&S
- Arterial blood gas:
  - Metabolic acidosis
- Raised lactate (may not be raised in chronic ischaemia)

⤢ AXR/erect CXR

⤢ CT/MR angiography

Treatment

⤢ IV fluids and resuscitation

⤢ Analgesia

⤢ Urinary catheter

⤢ Critical care input if unstable

⤢ NBM

⤢ NG tube

⤢ May require IV antibiotics

Further management

⤢ Depends on the cause and nature of presentation

⤢ Nonocclusive chronic ischaemia may be amenable to intra-arterial papaverine or anticoagulation

⤢ If acute ischaemia or evidence of bowel necrosis/perforation—urgent laparotomy

Chapter 17 **Breast pathology**

17.1 Benign breast disease

Fibroadenoma

- ↗ A benign overgrowth of one lobule of the breast
- ↗ Commonly occur in patients under the age of 30
- ↗ Painless, mobile, discrete lump
- ↗ Usually lobulated
- ↗ Diagnosed with USS/excision if unsure

Cysts

- ↗ Round symmetrical lump, may be discrete or multiple
- ↗ Aspiration of green-yellow fluid usually confirms diagnosis
- ↗ Can recur
- ↗ Mammography/USS needed if lump persists

Fibrocystic disease

- ↗ Combination of fibrosis, cyst formation, and inflammation
- ↗ Occurs between 15 and 55 years of age
- ↗ Characteristic cyclical pain and swelling
- ↗ Requires triple assessment
- ↗ Malignant transformation may occur

Intraductal papilloma

- ↗ Common in women 30–50 years of age
- ↗ Usually have blood-stained nipple discharge
- ↗ May have small palpable lump
- ↗ May not show on mammography, therefore requires galactogram if suspected ± biopsy
- ↗ Can be surgically excised

17.2 Breast carcinoma

Commonest cancer among women, affecting approximately 1 in 12.

Risk factors

- ↗ Age
- ↗ Nulliparity
- ↗ Early menarche/late menopause
- ↗ Previous history/family history
- ↗ *BRCA1* and *BRCA2* gene carrier
- ↗ Oral contraceptive pill
- ↗ Hormone replacement therapy

Histology and classification

- ↗ Noninvasive:
  - • Ductal CIS
  - • Lobular CIS

- Invasive:
  - Invasive ductal carcinoma
  - Invasive lobular carcinoma
- Mucinous
- Medullary
- Papillary
- Tubular

Investigations

- Clinical examination
- Mammography (if >50 years)
- USS (if <50 years)
- Fine needle aspiration cytology
- Trucut biopsy
- Excision biopsy
- Wire-guided biopsy
- CXR, bone scan, CT, MRI (to assess metastatic spread)

Triple assessment
1. Clinical examination
2. USS or mammography
3. Cytology/biopsy

'Red flag' examination findings

- Hard lump
- Fixation to surrounding structures
- Skin tethering
- Palpable axillary nodes
- Ulceration
- Nipple changes

6 D's of nipple changes
- Discoloration
- Discharge
- Depression
- Deviation
- Displacement
- Destruction

Staging

- TNM staging

Metastases

⌐ Direct invasion

⌐ Lymphatic spread

⌐ Lung, liver, brain, ovary, bone

Treatment

Surgical

⌐ Mastectomy

⌐ Wide local excision

⌐ Sentinel lymph node biopsy ± axillary lymph node clearance

Adjuvant or palliative

⌐ Hormonal

- Selective oestrogen receptor modulator (SERM), e.g. tamoxifen
- Aromatase inhibitor, e.g. anastrozole
- LHRH agonist
- Ovarian ablation

⌐ Chemotherapy

⌐ Radiotherapy

Section 3 Clinical

Chapter 18 **Common abdominal cases**

18.1 Hernia

This is a very common case for a physical examination station. You should be confident when examining these patients and have an understanding of the underlying anatomy, management, and potential complications of these conditions.

Examination

Inspect	• Scars/lump/distension • Ask the patient to cough or stand to reveal any hernia
Palpate	Abdomen and hernial orifices
Test	Cough impulse
Attempt reduction of hernia	If inguinal then attempt to differentiate direct from indirect
Also	Examine the scrotum

Present

'This is a 34-year-old man presents with a lump in his right groin, which originates above and medial to the pubic tubercle. On palpation it is soft, nontender, and reducible with a positive cough impulse. The scrotum is not involved and there is no evidence of a contralateral hernia. I am unable to contain the hernia with pressure over the deep ring, which implies that this is a reducible direct inguinal hernia.'

Likely questions

1. What is the definition of a hernia?

A hernia is a protrusion of a viscus or part of a viscus though the wall that normally contains it.

2. What conditions predispose to this condition?

↗ Cigarette smoking

↗ COPD

↗ Heavy manual work

↗ Previous surgery

3. What are the differential diagnosis for a lump in the groin?

↗ Hernia—inguinal or femoral

↗ Lymph nodes

↗ Saphena varix

↗ Ectopic testis

↗ Femoral aneurysm

↗ Psoas abscess

↗ Hydrocele of spermatic cord

↗ Lipoma

4. What are the boundaries of the inguinal canal?

The inguinal canal is a 4-cm channel that extends inferomedially from the deep to the superficial ring. Its boundaries are:

Roof	Arching fibres of internal oblique and transversus abdominis
Floor	Inguinal ligament
Anterior	External oblique aponeurosis, reinforced laterally by internal oblique
Posterior	Transversalis fascia, reinforced medial third by conjoint tendon

Internal ring Opening in the transversalis fascia

External ring Opening in the external oblique aponeurosis

5. What are the contents of the inguinal canal?

In women, the round ligament and genital branch of the genitofemoral nerve.

In men, the spermatic cord which consists of:

⤢ Three arteries:

- Artery to vas deferens
- Testicular artery
- Cremasteric artery

⤢ Three nerves:

- Ilioinguinal nerve
- Genitofemoral nerve
- Autonomic nerves

⤢ Three other structures:

- Vas deferens
- Pampiniform plexus of veins
- Lymphatics

6. What is the difference between an indirect and direct hernia?

An **indirect hernia** is usually congenital as it enters the inguinal canal through the deep ring. Clinically it may be controlled once reduced by pressure over the deep ring and during surgery is found to lie lateral to the inferior epigastric artery.

A **direct hernia** is more commonly acquired as it enters through the posterior wall of the inguinal canal at Hesselbach's triangle. In theory the hernia cannot be controlled by pressure over the deep ring and at surgery is found to lie medial to the inferior epigastric artery.

7. What are the boundaries of Hesselbach's triangle?

Laterally   Inferior epigastric artery

Medially   Rectus abdominus muscle

Inferiorly   Inguinal ligament

8. How can hernias be treated?

⤢ Conservatively, including treatment of underlying condition, i.e. COPD

⤢ Surgically, by mesh repair or direct repair

9. What are the complications of inguinal hernia repair?

Along with general complications associated with any surgical procedure, for this procedure I would specifically warn the patient about the risk of:

⤢ Urinary retention

⤢ Recurrence

⤢ Haematoma

⤢ Ongoing pain

⤢ Ischaemic orchitis

10. What are the boundaries of the femoral ring?

Anterior   Inguinal ligament

Medial   Lacunar ligament

Posterior   Pectineal ligament

Lateral   Femoral vein

> Femoral hernias are commoner in women but are still rarer than inguinal hernias. They have a higher incidence of strangulation and are usually repaired electively.
>
> **Remember:** on examination they originate below and lateral to the pubic tubercle.

11. What are the contents of the femoral sheath?

↗ Femoral artery laterally

↗ Femoral vein

↗ Femoral canal containing lymphatics medially

12. Why is strangulation more common in femoral hernias?

Strangulation is more common as three boundaries of the femoral ring are ligaments and the neck of the hernia is therefore narrower.

13. What surgical approaches are there to these hernias?

Classically there are three approaches to femoral hernia repair; whichever is used, the principle of surgery remain the same. These principles are to dissect the sac, reduce the contents, ligate the sac, and approximate the inguinal and pectineal ligaments.

↗ Infrainguinal (Lockwood's)—common in the elective setting

↗ Transinguinal (Lotheissen's)

↗ High approach (McEvedy's)—emergency procedure

14. What factors predispose to incisional hernia?

When answering this type of question you may find it useful to categorize your answer:

↗ Preoperative:

- Age
- Immunocompromised state (diabetes, steroids)
- Obesity
- Abdominal distension
- Malnutrition
- Cardiopulmonary disease

↗ Operative:

- Poor surgical technique
- Poor incision placement

↗ Postoperative:

- Wound haematoma
- Wound infection
- Early mobilization
- Chest infection and atelectasis

15. What are the treatment options?

This is commonly conservative as not all patients are suitable for surgery. In surgical repair, most incisional hernias require mesh repair.

18.2 Surgical jaundice

You may be confronted with a jaundiced patient and asked either to take a history or to examine the patient before discussing your likely management. Surgically the most important causes are those of obstructive jaundice and you should be confident discussing issues surrounding management of these patients.

Examination

⤢ History:
- Loss of weight or appetite
- History of gallstones or biliary operations
- Foreign travel, blood transfusion, alcohol intake

⤢ Inspection:
- Jaundice
- Signs of chronic liver disease

Jaundice is caused by an increase in the circulating bilirubin and becomes obvious clinically in the sclera when levels exceed 50 μmol/L.

⤢ Palpate:
- Hepatomegaly
- Hepatic masses
- Virchow's node

Remember **Courvoisier's law**: in the presence of obstructive jaundice, a mass in the right upper quadrant is unlikely to be due to gallstones.

Present

'This 74-year-old woman can be seen to be clinically jaundiced from the end of the bed. She has palmar erythema but no lymphadenopathy. Her abdomen is soft, with a palpable mass in her right upper quadrant, and there are no signs of ascites clinically. These findings are of obstructive jaundice and they would raise concerns of a malignant cause.'

Likely questions

1. How do you classify jaundice?

(This is a classic question and should be answered by classification into three groups; you should be able to recall a few common conditions for each group.)

Prehepatic   Haemolysis, spherocystosis, Gilbert's syndrome

Hepatic   Hepatitis, cirrhosis, drugs, toxins

Posthepatic   Gallstones, pancreatic carcinoma

2. What investigations would you consider in posthepatic jaundice?

⤢ Do not forget to mention blood tests
⤢ Abdominal USS
⤢ ERCP, CT scan, or MRCP may be appropriate

3. What are the specific complications of surgery in jaundiced patients?

Coagulopathy	Largely due to failure to absorb vitamin K from the gut
Hepatorenal syndrome	Mechanism unclear, but these patients should be well hydrated
Cholangitis	Severe complication that needs urgent management; causes Charcot's triad of rigors, abdominal pain, and jaundice

18.3 Stomas

A stoma is a surgically created communication between a hollow viscus and the skin. This is a common case seen on the examination station and it is therefore vital to have a grasp of the basics and be confident discussing issues relating to stoma care.

Examination

Inspect	• Site of the stoma • Other scars
Stomal appearance	Mucosal lining, spout, end or loop
Contents of the bag	Urine, loose or formed stool
Palpate	Offer to digitally palpate stoma (but this will not happen in the exam)

Present

'This 56-year-old man has a midline laparotomy scar as well as a stoma sited in his left iliac fossa. The stoma appears pink and healthy, and is flush with the skin. The stoma bag contains soft faeces. On palpation the abdomen is soft with no masses and there is no sign of any incisional or parastomal hernias. These findings are consistent with a healthy and functioning colostomy with evidence of previous laparotomy.'

Likely questions

1. What are the indications for a stoma?
 ↗ Feeding
 ↗ Diversion
 ↗ Lavage
 ↗ Exteriorization
 ↗ Decompression

2. What are the complications of a stoma?
 ↗ Ischaemia/gangrene
 ↗ Retraction
 ↗ Prolapse
 ↗ Parastomal hernia
 ↗ Stenosis
 ↗ Skin excoriation

3. How can you differentiate the types of stoma?

Site	Ileostomy more common in right iliac fossa (RIF), colostomy in left iliac fossa (LIF)
Surface	Ileostomy formed with a spout, colostomy flush with skin
Contents	Ileostomy has watery content, colostomy feculent

18.4 Enterocutaneous fistula

Examination

Inspect
- General condition
- Central lines for feedings
- Scars, stomas, drains, and site
- Content of discharge

Present

'On inspection this 34-year-old man has a stoma in his right iliac fossa, midline laparotomy scar, and midline opening covered by a stoma bag. He also has a Hickman line *in situ*. The stoma has a healthy spout and has watery contents. The midline defect has surrounding erythema and the bag contains similar watery contents. His abdomen is soft and nontender with no palpable masses. These findings are suggestive of an enterocutaneous fistula which may have been managed by ileostomy formation and TPN feeding.'

Likely questions

1. What is the definition of fistula?

An abnormal connection between two epithelial lined surfaces.

2. What is the aetiology of enterocutaneous fistula?

- Inflammation
- Radiotherapy
- Surgery
- Malignancy
- Trauma

3. Can you define the terms 'high-level fistula' and 'high-output fistula'?

A **high-level fistula** involves bowel at or above the ileum, whereas a low fistula originates from the large intestine.

A **high-output fistula** produces over 500 mL/ day and can lead to dehydration, electrolyte imbalance, and malnutrition.

4. What features are associated with unfavourable spontaneous closure?

Remember the mnemonic '**FRIEND**':

- **F**oreign body
- **R**adiation
- **I**nflammation/infection
- **E**pithelialization
- **N**eoplasm
- **D**istal obstruction

5. What are the principles of treatment?

- Skin protection
- Delineate the anatomy
- Control sepsis
- Relieve distal obstruction

⤷ Nutritional support

⤷ Correct fluid and electrolytes

18.5 Splenomegaly

Examination

A useful way to remember facts about the spleen is by using the numbers 1, 3, 5, 7, 9, 11:

⤷ The dimensions of the spleen are 1 × 3 × 5 inches (2.5 × 7.5 × 12.5 cm)

⤷ It weighs 7 ounces (~200 g)

⤷ It lies between the 9th and 11th ribs under the left diaphragm

When examining these patients there may not be other positive findings, but look out for associated hepatomegaly, anaemia, lymphadenopathy, or signs of rheumatoid arthritis.

Present

'On examination this 72-year-old man is comfortable at rest. He has cervical lymphadenopathy but there are no other positive peripheral signs. His abdomen is soft but there is a palpable mass extending from the left costal margin towards the umbilicus. I am unable to get above this mass, which moves on respiration and has a palpable notch. There are no signs of hepatomegaly or ascites. These findings are suggestive of splenomegaly, for which he requires further investigations.'

Likely questions

1. What features define splenomegaly on examination?

⤷ Cannot palpate above it

⤷ Moves with respiration

⤷ Cannot be balloted

⤷ A notch might be palpable

⤷ Extends down towards the umbilicus

2. What are the causes of splenomegaly?

This can be classified according to either aetiology or degree of enlargement:

⤷ Mild:
  • Polycythaemia rubra vera
  • Haemolytic anaemias
  • Infective causes

⤷ Moderate:
  • Portal hypertension
  • Lymphoma/leukaemias

⤷ Massive:
  • Myelofibrosis
  • Malaria
  • Chronic Myeloid Leukaemia

3. What are the indications for splenectomy?

⤷ Trauma

⤷ Hypersplenism, i.e. haemolytic anaemia, spherocytosis, sickle cell disease, myelofibrosis

4. What specific precautions do you need to take after splenectomy?

Usually postsplenectomy prophylaxis includes:

↗ Vaccination against pneumococcus, *Haemophilus influenzae*, and meningococcus

↗ Lifelong penicillin prophylaxis

↗ Annual influenza vaccination

18.6 Hepatomegaly

Examination

Inspect • Jaundice
• Hands—clubbing, palmar erythema, Dupuytren's, liver flap
• Trunk—gynaecomastia, loss of axillary hair, >5 spider naevi

Palpate • Hepatomegaly (degree of enlargement and the liver edge)
• Liver nodules
• Ascites

Present

'This 68-year-old woman is comfortable at rest. On inspection she is cachectic with palmar erythema but there are no signs of clubbing or lymphadenopathy. Her abdomen is soft and she is mildly tender in the right upper quadrant where there is a firm and irregular palpable liver edge that extends 2 cm below the costal margin. There are no signs clinically of ascites or splenomegaly. These findings are suspicious of a malignant cause for her hepatomegaly which would require further investigation.'

Likely questions

1. What are the commonest causes of hepatomegaly?

↗ Liver metastases

↗ Alcoholic liver disease

↗ Myelofibrosis

↗ Right side cardiac failure

↗ Hepatocellular carcinoma

2. How would you investigate a patient with hepatomegaly?

After a full history and examination I would request:

↗ Bloods—FBC, liver function, clotting, 'liver screen'

↗ USS first line radiological test

↗ Contrast CT

3. What is portal hypertension?

A raised portal vein pressure (>10 mmHg) which results in reduced blood flow. Defined as abnormal interstitial fluid accumulation in the peritoneal cavity; on examination this is elicited by 'shift in dullness' or 'fluid thrill'. Its causes can be divided into:

Extrahepatic Portal or splenic vein thrombosis

Intrahepatic Cirrhosis, right heart failure

18.7 Ascites

Examination

Inspect • Abdominal distension
• Hands—looking for signs of chronic liver disease

Palpate
- Organomegaly (remember to percuss as palpation can be difficult in presence of gross ascites)
- 'Shifting dullness'
- 'Fluid thrill'
- Generalized oedema (ankles and sacrum)

Present

'This 53-year-old man has gross abdominal distension. On inspection he has finger clubbing, palmar erythema, and a liver flap but there are no signs of peripheral oedema. His abdomen is soft and I am unable to palpate or percuss any organomegaly. However, on percussion there is shift in dullness. These findings are suggestive of ascites, which is likely to be hepatic in origin.'

Remember: ascitic fluid with>30 g/L protein is an **exudate** and <30 g/L is a **transudate**.

Likely questions

1. What are the causes of ascites?

Answer by dividing causes into transudates and exudates:

↗ Transudates:
- Chronic liver disease
- Cardiac failure
- Renal failure
- Hypoalbuminaemia

↗ Exudates:
- Intra-abdominal malignancy
- Infection
- Lymphatic obstruction

2. How would you perform an ascitic tap?

In a consented and appropriately prepared patient I would:

↗ Lie the patient supine and percuss/mark the transition from dull to resonant

↗ Infiltrate local anaesthetic

↗ Aspitate

↗ Send fluid for cytology, biochemistry, and microbiology

18.8 Abdominal aortic aneurysm

Examination

Inspect
- Scars
- Pulsating masses (unlikely!)

Palpate
- Superficial and deep palpation as normal
- Palpate with both hands for presence of aneurysm and estimate size
- Offer to palpate other lower limb pulses and check for distal aneurysms

Remember: aorta bifurcates at L4 so don't palpate too low.

Auscultate Listen over aorta and iliacs for bruits

Present

'This 86-year-old man is comfortable at rest with no positive findings on inspection. His abdomen is soft and nontender with a pulsatile mass in the midline of around 5 cm with no bruits. All his lower limb pulses are present bilaterally. These findings are suggestive of an abdominal aortic aneurysm of around 5 cm in size and this patient would warrant further investigation.'

Likely questions

1. What is the definition of an aneurysm?

An abnormal dilatation of a blood vessel; in the aorta the diameter is >3 cm.

2. What are the complications of the aneurysm?

⤢ Rupture

⤢ Thrombosis

⤢ Embolism

⤢ Pressure on adjacent structures

⤢ Fistula into adjacent structures

3. What are the options for management?

Options include surveillance and operative repair, which can be done either as an open procedure or endovascularly. Ultrasound scans are useful in monitoring the size of the aneurysm but preoperatively CT scan may be used to identify the exact location of the aneurysm and the involvement of the renal arteries. When deciding on surgical intervention important factors to consider are the size of the aneurysm (if >5.5 cm then elective repair is recommended), whether it is symptomatic, the rate of growth, and the patient's age and comorbidities.

18.9 Scrotal lumps

This is a common condition to come across in your practical station. You will need to look comfortable examining the patient and hold a discussion about the likely differentials.

Examination

Inspect	• Does the swelling arise from scrotum or groin?
	• Look for surgical incisions in the groin or median raphe
Palpate	• Testes and describe lumps
	• Can you get above the lump?
	• Is the lump separate from the testis and epididymis?
Tests	• Does it transilluminate?
Also	• Offer to examine the groin

Present

'This 25-year-old man has a swelling of his right testicle. On palpation I am able to get above the lump which is 2 × 3 cm, hard, and inseparable from the testis itself. The lump does not transilluminate, the other testis is normal, and there are no signs of hernias or inguinal lymphadenopathy. These findings suggest the swelling is testicular in origin and raise suspicions of a testicular tumour.'

Likely questions

1. What is the differential of a scrotal lump?

⤢ Hydrocele

⤢ Varicocele

⤢ Epididymal cyst

⤢ Hernia

⤢ Testicular carcinoma

⤢ Epididymitis

2. What is a hydrocele and what are the different types?

Hydrocele is defined as a fluctuant and transilluminable swelling that cannot be felt separate to the testis, it is caused by an abnormal quantity of fluid within the tunica vaginalis. Typically four different types are described:

Vaginal hydrocele	Obliteration of processus vaginalis with fluid around testis only
Hydrocele of the cord	Fluid only in cord
Congenital hydrocele	Patent processus vaginalis and communication between tunica and peritoneal cavity
Infantile hydrocele	Obliteration of processus near deep ring

3. Define a varicocele. What symptoms may it cause?

A varicocele is the presence of dilated and tortuous veins in the pampiniform plexus. Although they are usually asymptomatic, patients may complain of a dragging sensation or they can be associated with subfertility. They are more common on the left side, where the testicular vein drains directly into the renal vein, which is why their sudden appearance in a middle-aged man should raise suspicion of renal cancer.

4. What are the typical findings of a testicular tumour on examination?

Typically on examination a hard, irregular swelling which is inseparable from the testis is felt. There may be an associated secondary hydrocele.

5. What types of testicular tumour are most common?

They are the commonest solid tumours in the 25–35 year age group and the main types are seminomas and teratomas.

Remember: orchidectomies are performed via an inguinal approach to prevent involvement of the scrotum, which has a separate lymphatic drainage.

Chapter 19 Common thoracic cases

19.1 Pleural effusion

Examination

Inspect	• Cyanosis
	• Tachypnoea
	• Unequal chest expansion
Palpate	Diminished tactile fremitus
Percuss	Dull to percussion
Auscultate	• Reduced air entry
	• Reduced vocal resonance

Present

'This 63-year-old woman looks tachypnoeic at rest with minimal movement from right side of chest wall. The percussion note is dull on the right base with diminished tactile fremitus. On auscultation the air entry is reduced, as is vocal resonance at the right base. These clinical findings are consistent with a pleural effusion which could be confirmed through further investigations.'

Likely questions

1. How would you classify pleural effusions and their causes?

Pleural effusions are classified according to protein content as either exudates (>30 mg/L) or transudates (<30 mg/L).

↗ Causes of transudate:

- Heart failure
- Liver cirrhosis
- Nephritic syndrome

↗ Causes of exudate:

- Neoplastic
- Infection
- Pulmonary embolism
- Trauma
- Pancreatitis

2. What are the indications for placing a chest drain?

↗ Pneumothorax, or chest injury if patient ventilated

↗ Tension pneumothorax or persistent after aspiration

↗ Malignant pleural effusion

↗ Empyema

↗ Traumatic haemopneumothorax

↗ Post thoracotomy, oesophagectomy, or cardiac surgery

3. How would you safely insert a chest drain?

Firstly, I would ensure the patient is properly consented, locally anaethetized, positioned and prepped. Then:

↗ Get equipment ready, ensuring a drain with underwater seal is available

↗ Confirm the side on examination and radiograph, and sit the patient at 45°

↗ Safest entry point is the 5th intercostal space in the midaxillary line

⤢ Make stab incision, deepen with blunt dissection, insert finger to ensure lung not adherent

⤢ Use a haemostat to insert drain, connect to underwater seal, suture drain in place

⤢ Don't forget to request a check radiograph

Remember: the intercostal bundle runs inferior to each rib.

19.2 Pneumothorax

A pneumothorax is defined as the accumulation of air in the pleural space due to either disruption of visceral or parietal pleura.

Examination

Inspect	• Cyanosis
	• Tachypnoea
	• Tachycardia
	• Unequal chest expansion
Palpation	Trachea central
Percuss	Hyper-resonant percussion note
Auscultate	• Breath sounds absent or decreased
	• Reduced vocal resonance

Remember: trachea is deviated only in massive or tension pneumothorax.

Present

'This is a 30-year-old man who is tachypnoeic at rest with a respiratory rate of 30 and reduced chest wall movement on his left side. His trachea is central with hyper-resonance over the entire left side. The breath sounds are absent and vocal resonance reduced. These findings are consistent with a pneumothorax which could be confirmed with a chest radiograph.'

Likely questions

1. What are the different types of pneumothoraces?

Spontaneous	• Occurs without trauma
	• **Primary**—without underlying chest condition
	• **Secondary**—with an underlying chest pathology
Traumatic	Blunt or penetrating thoracic trauma
Iatrogenic	Postoperative, central venous catheter insertion, mechanical ventilation
Tension	Pneumothorax with tissue forming a valve allowing air to enter pleural space, but not to leave

2. How would you manage a simple pneumothorax?

A small pneumothorax in a healthy individual does not necessarily require treatment, although aspiration may be attempted. More commonly a chest drain may be required if:

⤢ Large pneumothorax with dyspnoea

⤢ Pneumothorax in association with a pre-existing lung disease

⤢ Pneumothorax which is increasing in size

⤢ Not self-resolving in 1 week

3. Define the term 'tension pneumothorax'. What clinical signs would you expect?

A tension pneumothorax occurs when air accumulates in the pleural space through a one-way valve with the pneumothorax enlarging with every breath and causing mediastinal displacement. On examination you would find an unwell patient who is extremely tachypnoeic and tachycardic. On inspection there would be unequal chest expansion and the trachea would be deviated away from the affected side. There would be hyper-resonance and diminished or absent breath sounds on the affected side. It is an immediately life-threatening condition requiring immediate decompression.

4. What are the management steps for a tension pneumothorax?

The first step is recognition of the condition; these patients should be diagnosed and treated clinically before they have any radiography.

A structured answer here using the 'ABC' is acceptable but you should stress the urgent need to decompress with a large cannula inserted into the 2nd intercostal space at the midclavicular line.

The second step is insertion of a chest drain as described previously for pleural effusion (Question 3 above).

19.3 Thoracotomy scars

Examination

Inspect • General condition
• Presence of chest drains or scars
• Chest expansion

Palpate Tracheal position, deviated in pneumonectomy

Percuss Hyper-resonant on side with remaining lung, dull on pneumonectomy side

Present

'This 70-year-old woman is comfortable at rest and has a lateral thoracotomy scar. Her respiratory rate is 16 but there is minimal expansion of the right side of her chest. The trachea is deviated to the right where there is hyper-resonance and harsh breath sounds. The finding is that this patient had undergone previous pulmonary surgery such as a pneumonectomy.'

Likely questions

1. What surgical approaches are you aware of to access the thorax?

Posterolateral thoracotomy	Runs from midway between medial border of scapula and vertebral spinous processes before extending in line of a rib below the tip of scapula to midaxillary line
Midline sternotomy	Incision runs from 1 cm below suprasternal notch to 6 cm below xiphisternum
Anterior thoracotomy	Runs in line with ribs anteriorly
Right parasternal	Vertical incision lateral to sternum which involves dislocation of costosternal junctions

2. What typical procedures are performed through a midline sternotomy?

↗ Coronary artery bypass surgery

↗ Aortic or mitral valve replacement

3. What typical procedures are performed through a posterolateral thoracotomy?

↗ Nodule resection

↗ Lobectomy

↗ Pneumonectomy

↗ Oesophageal surgery

↗ Thoracic spinal surgery

19.4 Dextrocardia

In the past this case has turned up in OSCE stations and has been known to catch candidates off guard. It is therefore worth keeping the possibility of dextrocardia in the back of your mind.

Examination

Inspect	• Scars
	• Peripheral cardiac signs
	• Jugular venous pressure
Palpate	• Pulse and volume
	• Positioned apex beat
Auscultate	• Heart sounds
	• Lung bases

Present

'This 32-year-old woman is comfortable at rest. Her pulse is 80, regular, and of good volume. The jugular venous pressure is not visible. The apex beat is palpable only on the right side of the chest at the 5th intercostal space in the midclavicular line. Her heart sounds are heard with no additional sounds. These findings are consistent with dextrocardia.'

Likely questions

1. What other examination would you perform, and why?

Once you have examined the cardiovascular system you should offer to examine the abdomen and respiratory system. This is done to look for evidence of situs inversus or Kartagener's syndrome, which are associated with dextrocardia.

2. What is Kartagener's syndrome?

This is a syndrome where a patient suffers from dextrocardia, bronchiectasis, situs inversus, infertility, dysplasia of frontal sinuses, sinusitis, and otitis media.

3. What is situs inversus?

In situs inversus the viscera of thorax and abdomen are found on the opposite side from the normal anatomical position. The patient is usually asymptomatic.

19.5 Carcinoma

Bronchial carcinoma is the commonest cancer in men and the second commonest in women. Only surgical resection offers hope of long-term survival, but at presentation most patients have inoperable disease and treatment involves a combination of radiotherapy, chemotherapy, and palliation.

Examination

Inspect	• General condition
	• Hands for cyanosis, clubbing, nicotine staining, and CO_2 flap
	• Equal chest expansion
Palpatate	• Tracheal position
	• Lymphadenopathy

Present

'On inspection this 84-year-old man is cachetic, with both nicotine staining and finger clubbing. There is equal expansion of the chest wall with a centrally positioned trachea. On auscultation there is reduced air entry over the left upper zone with a monophonic wheeze.'

Likely questions

1. What are the four types of lung carcinoma?

⤳ Adenocarcinoma (40%)

⤳ Squamous cell carcinoma (30%)

⤳ Large-cell undifferentiated carcinoma (25%)

⤳ Small-cell carcinoma (5%)

2. What is a Pancoast's tumour?

This is an apical lung tumour which can cause compression of the brachiocephalic vein, subclavian artery, phrenic nerve, 1st thoracic spinal nerve, recurrent laryngeal nerve, or sympathetic ganglion. Sympathetic ganglion compression can cause miosis, anhidrosis, ptosis, and enopthalmos, which collectively are known as **Horner's syndrome**.

3. With which paraneoplastic syndromes is lung carcinoma typically associated?

Lung carcinoma can be associated with the release of antidiuretic hormone (SIADH), adrenocortico-tropic hormone, or parathyroid hormone related protein.

4. How might you assess a patient's suitability for surgical treatment?

When answering this question you should categorize your answer into patient and tumour factors:

⤳ Patient factors:

- Exercise tolerance
- Medical history
- Signs of secondaries
- Investigate using lung function test (FEV_1 >1.5 L and FEV_1/FVC ratio >50% indicate that pneumonectomy would be feasible)

⤳ Tumour factors:

- Staging using CT and/or PET scan
- Mediastinoscopy to evaluate mediastinal lymph nodes if appear enlarged

19.6 Valvular heart disease

Examination

Inspect	• Scars
	• High arch palate and malar flush
	• Raised jugular venous pressure
Palpate	• Pulses (slow-rising/collapsing)
	• Apex beat
	• Heaves and thrills
Auscultate	• Heart sounds
	• Additional sounds/murmurs—timing, site, radiation
	• Lung bases

Present

'This 57-year-old woman on inspection is comfortable at rest. She has a regular slow-rising pulse of 72 and the apex is displaced to the anterior axillary line in the 6th intercostal space. The 1st and 2nd heart sounds are present, with an ejection systolic murmur that radiates to the neck. The lung bases are clear. These findings are consistent with aortic stenosis.'

Likely questions

1. What are the common types of valve pathology and their associated murmurs and clinical signs?

↗ Aortic regurgitation:
- Causes include rheumatic heart disease, endocarditis, Marfan's syndrome, syphilis, and dissection
- Early diastolic murmur
- Collapsing pulse

↗ Aortic stenosis:
- Caused by congenital bicuspid valves or rheumatic heart disease
- Mid systolic murmur, radiates to neck
- Slow-rising pulse
- May see signs of left ventricular hypertrophy

↗ Mitral regurgitation:
- Caused by rheumatic fever and myocardial infarction
- Pansystolic murmur
- Can be associated with atrial fibrillation

↗ Mitral stenosis:
- Caused by rheumatic fever or cardiac infections
- Heard best at apex
- Diastolic murmur
- Associated with malar flush

↗ Pulmonary stenosis:
- Cause usually congenital
- Ejection systolic murmur

2. What two types of heart valves can be inserted?

↗ Metallic heart valves:
- Patient less likely to require reoperation
- Will need lifelong anticoagulation with warfarin

↗ Tissue heart valves:
- Currently human or porcine valves used
- Eventual degeneration of the heart valve with need to reoperation
- Anticoagulation is not required

3. What issues are important in the perioperative management of metallic heart valves?

The patient's medical history should be made available to the anaesthetist including ECGs, current exercise tolerance, current medications, and recent echocardiogram to ensure the patient is optimized for surgery.

The patients' anticoagulation will have to be stopped preoperatively. The usual practice is to convert the patient on to an intravenous heparin infusion while their INR is subtherapeutic. This infusion has the advantage of having a shorter half-life and aims to keep the patient off anticoagulation for the shortest time possible.

Patients with valve abnormalities undergoing surgical procedures are at risk of infective endocarditis, and local guidelines should be followed regarding antibiotic prophylaxis.

4. What is the New York Heart Association classification relating to heart disease?

This is a scoring system used to assess the severity of symptoms and the effect of cardiac disease on patients' quality of life:

Class I   No limitation on any activities

Class II   Mild limitation of activities with symptoms produced on exertion

Class III   Marked limitation of activities, only comfortable at rest

Class IV   Symptoms present at rest and worsened on any exertion

19.7 Preoperative station

A common scenario is to be asked to attend the preoperative clinic because a member of the nursing staff has raised concerns over a particular patient. In the past this station has involved the candidate being required to examine the patient and interpret ECGs before discussing issues relating to pre- and perioperative management of the patient.

Examination

Inspect	• General condition
	• Scars
	• Jugular venous pressure
Palpate	• Pulse—rate, rhythm, and volume
	• Position of apex beat
Auscultate	• Heart sounds
	• Additional sounds and murmurs
	• Lung bases

Presentation

'This 68-year-old woman is comfortable at rest. There is a scar over the upper left half of the chest wall. Her pulse is 60 beats per minute and is regular. Her jugular venous pressure could not be visualized and the apex can be felt in the 5th intercostal space in the midclavicular line. The 1st and 2nd heart sounds are heard with no additional sounds and the lung bases are clear. These findings could be suggestive of a patient with a permanent pacemaker.'

Likely questions

1. What does this ECG show?

You may well be expected to interpret ECGs during your examination and therefore you should be competent in interpreting commonly occurring cases. Examples include atrial fibrillation, paced rhythm, or myocardial infarction.

2. What preoperative issues are there with a patient with a permanent pacemaker?

Before the patient can safely undergo an elective procedure it is necessary to:

↗ Inform the anaesthetist

↗ Ask the patient of any recent symptoms of syncope, shortness of breath, or palpitations

↗ Check exactly which type of pacemaker the patient has

↗ Arrange pacemaker servicing if this has not been done recently

↗ Ask about cardiac medications, especially anticoagulants

3. What intraoperative problems can you foresee, and how would you prepare yourself for these?

Problems can be avoided if the above information has been gathered at an early stage and the multi-disciplinary team informed. The main concern would be the use of diathermy: ideally the diathermy pad should be sited away from the heart and the surgeon should use bipolar if possible. It would also be worth having the equipment for temporary pacing available, in case a problem with the pacemaker occurred during the procedure.

4. What preoperative issues do you foresee in a patient with atrial fibrillation?

If the atrial fibrillation is new in onset, then the patient should have their atrial fibrillation optimized prior to an elective procedure. This will normally involve informing the general practitioner of the finding, with a subsequent cardiology opinion when required.

If the patient has established atrial fibrillation then you should review their regular medications (with specific mention to warfarin), ensuring that the condition is rate controlled, and that the patient is asymptomatic before proceeding.

5. How would you manage a patient on warfarin undergoing an elective procedure?

You would first need to establish the indication for warfarinization as this will affect the subsequent management. For example, patients with atrial fibrillation can:

↗ Have their warfarin stopped prior to admission

↗ Have their INR checked before surgery

↗ Be treated with prophylactic heparin while an inpatient

↗ Recommence warfarin when safe postoperatively

In contrast, patients with metallic heart valves will need to be admitted once their INR is subtherapeutic and started on intravenous heparin infusion. Similarly, this infusion will continue postoperatively until the INR is therapeutic.

In practice these patients are usually discussed with either the cardiologist or haematologist regarding the best anticoagulation regime.

PART 2
LIMBS AND SPINE

Section 1 Anatomy

Chapter 20 **Bones and joints**

It is a safe assumption for any candidate taking the MRCS that at least one 9-minute station will be based around bony specimens. Questions will be mainly focus on anatomy but may well also incorporate wider bone physiology and pathology.

The skeletal system serves as a site of attachment for muscles allowing movement, a site for haematopoiesis, a mineral store, and to protect organs. It consists of bones, joints, and associated connective tissues. A joint is an articulation between two or more bones. There are three main types: synovial, fibrous and cartilaginous.

20.1 Bone tissue

Bone is a dense connective tissue comprised of hydroxyapatite, a calcium/phosphate crystal structure, bound to a collagen matrix. Bone tissue is divided into two **types**, two **structures**, and two **forms.**

Two types

Woven bone

⤢ Disorganized and weak

⤢ Found in infants, callus, and tumours

Lamellar bone

⤢ Stronger and organized

⤢ Oriented to stress

⤢ Mature bone tissue

⤢ Occurs in cancellous and cortical bone

> **Remember:** all 'normal', adult bone is of lamellar **type** found arranged in either of the two cortical or cancellous **structures.**

Two structures

Cortical bone

⤢ 80% of bone tissue

⤢ Arranged in the **haversian system** of central canals containing blood vessels surrounded by concentric lamellae of bone

⤢ Found in the diaphysis (shaft) of bones

⤢ Metabolically less active

Cancellous bone

⤢ Lattice arrangement with marrow tissue interposed between **trabeculae**

⤢ Found at metaphysis

⤢ Metabolically more active than cortical bone, with constant remodelling

Two forms

Flat bones

⤢ E.g. bones of the skull and pelvis

⤢ Formed by intramembranous ossification

Long bones

⤢ E.g. femur and humerus

⤢ Have four parts:

- Epiphysis
- Physis
- Metaphysis
- Diaphysis

⤢ Formed by endochondral ossification

20.2 Bone formation and growth

Bone is formed in two ways: endochondral or intramembranous ossification.

Endochondral ossification

⤳ Bone tissue replaces a cartilage model

⤳ Occurs in long bone formation in embryo, at the physeal growth plates, and in fracture healing

Intramembranous ossification

⤳ Occurs without cartilage

⤳ Mesenchymal cells form layers of membranes and then differentiate into osteoblasts which then start to lay down bony tissue

20.3 Synovial joints

Structure

Synovial joints are the commonest type of joint in the body. A synovial joint is characterized by three features:

⤳ Articular capsule:

  • Lined with synovial membrane and continuous with the periosteum

  • Is avascular but highly innervated

  • Contains stretch receptors, key components of proprioception

⤳ Synovial membrane:

  • Produces the synovial fluid which lubricates the joint, allowing almost friction-less movement

  • Covers inside of joint capsule and all intra-articular surfaces except articular cartilage

⤳ Articular cartilage:

  • Hyaline cartilage that covers the areas of the bone epiphysis which articulate with the other bone

  • Reduces friction, absorbs impact, and spreads load

Classification

Synovial joints can be further divided according to structure or mechanism.

Structural types

Primary synovial joint	No meniscus, e.g. elbow joint (humerus–ulna)
Secondary synovial joint	Intra-articular meniscus which absorbs shock, distributes loads, and reduces friction, e.g. knee joint

Mechanical types

Hinge	Allows movement in only one plane, e.g. elbow joint (humerus–ulna)
Ball and socket	Capable of rotational movement, e.g. glenohumeral
Gliding	Allows sliding movements, e.g. radio-scaphoid joint
Pivot	One bone moves in more than one plane around another, e.g. knee
Condyloid	Each articular surface is nonconforming, giving rise to specialist movements, e.g. wrist
Saddle	A condyloid joint where one surface is saddle shaped, e.g. carpo-metacarpal joint of thumb (most common site of osteoarthritis in the hand)

20.4 Fibrous joints

Fibrous joints are characterized by the articulating bones being held together by strong fibrous tissue, which allow little movement. There are two main types:

Sutures	Joints between the bones of the skull that allow almost no movement and often undergo ossification
Syndesmosis	Joint between the distal long bones of the limbs i.e. the proximal and distal joints of the radius and ulna and the tibia and fibular which allow more movement than sutures and do not ossify

20.5 Cartilaginous joints

When the bones in a join articulate via intervening cartilaginous tissue, they are described as a **cartilaginous joint**. There are two types:

⤢ Primary cartilaginous joints:

- Bones are connected by cartilage
- May be thick **fibrocartilage**, allowing limited movement, e.g. acromioclavicular joint, or more flexible hyaline cartilage, e.g. costosternal joints

⤢ Secondary cartilaginous joints:

- Occur only in midline and also called **symphysis**
- Bone surfaces are covered by **hyaline cartilage**, like synovial joints
- Bones articulate with intervening fibrocartilage tissue, i.e. pubic symphysis and intervertebral discs

Chapter 21 **Spine**

As with the rest of the skeletal system the spine must be revised using a skeleton, as this is a likely way for the subject to be introduced in the exam. This chapter contains the key facts and concepts that the candidate should be able to articulate to the examiners.

The spinal canal is constructed from 33 vertebrae and their intervening vertebral discs arranged into a sinusoidal curve. Its functions are:

↗ To support the head and neck

↗ To protect the spinal cord and cauda equina

↗ To provide an attachment for muscles

↗ Haematopoiesis

21.1 Spinal regions

Cervical
- 7 vertebrae (but eight pairs of spinal nerves)
- **Lordotic** curve

Thoracic
- 12 vertebrae
- **Kyphotic** curve

Lumbar
- 5 vertebrae
- **Lordotic** curve
- Spinal cord becomes **cauda equina** at L1

Sacral 5 fused vertebrae part of pelvic ring

Coccyx 4 fused vestigial vertebrae (3–5)

21.2 Typical vertebrae

Vertebral body Weight-bearing component of spinal column

Neural arch
- Surrounds and protects the spinal cord
- Comprised of two **pedicles** arising from the vertebral body, meeting two **lamina** which complete the arch
- Gives off three processes; two **transverse process** which arise from the meeting of the pedicles and lamina and one **spinous process** which arises from the meeting of the two lamina

Intervertebral facet joints Synovial joints between consecutive vertebrae

Intervertebral foramen Not true a true foramen but the space between pedicles of consecutive vertebrae

Identifying a vertebra

Transverse foramen
- Transverse process of cervical vertebrae **only**
- Transmits vertebral arteries, veins, and sympathetic fibres

Costal facets
- Thoracic vertebrae **only**
- Articulate with ribs

> Identifying a vertebral bone is a question of determining whether it possesses the special features of either cervical or thoracic vertebrae. If it possesses neither, it must be either a lumbar vertebra, C1 (atlas), or C2 (axis)

21.3 Spinal ligaments

Anterior longitudinal ligament

↗ Lies on anterior surface of vertebral bodies from **occiput** to sacrum

↗ Resists hyperextension

Posterior longitudinal ligament
- ↗ Runs in vertebral canal, on posterior surface of vertebral bodies from C2 to sacrum
- ↗ Resists hyperextension

Ligamentum flavum
- ↗ Connects adjacent lamina
- ↗ Resists hyperflexion

Interspinous ligaments
- ↗ Runs between adjacent spinous process

Ligamentum nuchae
- ↗ Travels along tips of cervical spinous processes, between **occipital protuberance** and C7

21.4 Cervical spine

Key features

The seven cervical vertebrae are the smallest of the unfused vertebrae.

Considerable movement occurs at the cervical spine, mostly at the **axial-atlanto-**occipital joints.

Transverse foramina in transverse processes transmit vertebral vessels before they enter **cranial vault** via **foramen magnum.**

All have a **bifid spinous process** which is attached to ligamentum nuchae.

> Spinal nerve pairs C1–C7 are named relative to the vertebral body **below.** C7 has two pairs of nerves, C7 and C8. All thoracic, lumbar, and sacral spinal nerves are named in relation to the vertebral body **above.**

Typical cervical vertebrae (C3–C6)
- ↗ Vertebral body is small relative to foramen
- ↗ Intervertebral facet joints allow forward flexion/extension

C1 (atlas)
- ↗ No body (actually body fused with body of C2 to form **dens** or peg) but thin anterior arch
- ↗ No spinous process
- ↗ Broad superior facets articulate with **occipital condyles** for flexion/extension of skull on atlas: the **atlanto-occipital joint**
- ↗ Articular facet on inner surface of anterior arch, which forms synovial joint with dens
- ↗ Atlantal ring divided into anterior one-third (dens) and posterior two-thirds by **transverse atlantal ligament**

C2 (axis)
- ↗ No body, but dens formed from vertebral bodies of C1 and C2
- ↗ Broad superior articular facets allow gliding rotation of C1 around dens of C2 (atlanto-axial joint)

C7
- ↗ Transverse foramina variable (may be absent, divided into two, or transmit only **vertebral vein**, not artery, on one or both sides)
- ↗ Prominent nonbifid spinous process

21.5 Thoracic spine

Key features

↗ 12 thoracic vertebrae

↗ Little movement, only limited rotation due to splinting effect of thoracic cage

↗ Intervertebral facets almost vertical

↗ All have some kind of costal facet

↗ Relatively small vertebral foramen

Typical thoracic vertebrae (T2–T8)

↗ 'Heart-shaped' bodies

↗ 'Club shaped' transverse process

↗ Two pairs of **costocapitular demifacets** on vertebral body

↗ The upper facet articulates with the rib of the same vertebral level

↗ Facets on traverse process, which articulate with tubercles of corresponding rib (costotubercular facets)

T1

↗ Superior costocapitular facet is complete and not a demifacet

↗ Prominent spinous process, like C7

T9–T12

↗ Often only have one pair of costocapitular facets which are typically complete, not a demifacet

↗ T10–12 lack a costotubercular facet

↗ T12 similar in appearance to lumbar vertebrae

21.6 Lumbar spine

Key features

↗ Five lumbar vertebrae with neither costal facets nor transverse foramina

↗ Large body to foramen ratio

↗ Concave oblique intervertebral facets to allow forward and lateral flexion

↗ L1 contains **conus medularis** (end of cord) spinous and transverse processes, large and strong, allowing for their significant muscular attachments

↗ L5 often fused with sacrum

21.7 Sacrum and coccyx

Sacrum: key features

↗ Fused, inverted triangle shaped, component of pelvis

↗ Articulates with ilium via sacroiliac joints

↗ Articulates with L5 via L5/S1 disc and intervertebral facet joints

↗ Four pairs of pelvic and dorsal foramen that communicate with the sacral canal

↗ Dorsal median crest analogous to spinous processes. Sacral canal contains the distal **cauda equina**, and **filum terminale**, with spinal nerves S1–S4 leaving via the sacral foramen (ventral roots via pelvic foramen, dorsal roots via dorsal foramen)

↗ Dura ends at level of S2

↗ Both S5 nerves along with the filum terminale exit the sacral canal dorsally via the sacral hiatus

Coccyx: key features

↗ Small, fusion of four vertebrae, articulates with sacral apex

21.8 Joints in the spine

There are three groups of intervertebral joints in the spine:

↗ intervertebal discs (symphyses)

↗ facet joints (synovial joints)

↗ atlanto-axial joints (synovial joints)

Intervertebral discs

Inferior and superior surface of vertebral bodies, covered in hyaline cartilage.

Annulus fibrosus   Tough outer shell of disc; fibrocartilage and small amounts of collagen

Nucleus pulposus   Gelatinous at birth, but becomes increasingly like fibrocartilage with age

Disc prolapse occurs when nucleus pulposus herniates through damaged annulus fibrosus to press on spinal nerve roots (laterally) or cord/cauda equina (centrally).

Facet joints

↗ Simple synovial joints in cervical and thoracic spine

↗ Complex synovial joints in lumbar spine with **meniscoid** structures

Atlanto-axial joints

↗ Three synovial joints, consisting of the articulation between the dens and atlas and a pair of facet joints, all of which allow rotation

Chapter 22 **Osteology**

There is only one way to learn osteology: with an anatomy textbook and a skeleton. This chapter will teach you how to convert that knowledge into the form the examiners want.

Most candidates will be handed bony specimens during their exam. The format is predictable, with the candidate being asked to identify the specimen and the main bony features, and then being invited to talk about attachments and specific features. Each area will be the subject of about 2½ minutes of questioning.

When first handed the specimen, orient it anatomically, and point at features with a pointer or pen **systematically**, e.g. proximal to distally.

In these sample answers a * is used to indicate when you should be pointing, and key features you need to be confident of are in **bold**.

22.1 Shoulder girdle and humerus

Typical questions

1. **Identify this specimen and its key features and attachments**

This is a right shoulder, comprised of **clavicle***, **scapula***, and **humerus***. The shoulder actually consists of four joints: the **glenohumeral joint***, the **acromioclavicular** joint*, the **sternoclavicular joint,** and the articulation between the scapular and thoracic wall.

The proximal third of the clavicle serves as the site of attachment for **sternocleidomastoid***, and distally the **corococlavicular ligament** attaches to the **conoid tubercle***.

The posterior aspect of the scapula is divided into the **infra*-** and **supraspinous fossa*** by the **scapular spine*** and anteriorly lies the **subscapular fossa***. The spine continues as the **acromion***, anterior to which is the **corocoid***, which is the site of attachment of the **conjoint tendon.** The **glenoid*** is the articular surface between the scapular and the humerus.

The proximal humerus has a large articular surface* bordered by the **anatomical neck***. The **greater tuberosity*** is the site of insertion of the **supraspinatus muscle** and the **lesser tuberosity*** is the site of insertion of subscapularis. Between the two is the **intertubercular (bicipital) groove***, where the long head of biceps tendon resides. The **deltoid tuberosity*** is the site of attachment of deltoid. The **radial groove*** transmits the radial nerve distally.

> **Remember:** 'anatomy comes before surgery'—anatomical neck is proximal to surgical neck of humerus.

2. **You mentioned the glenohumeral joint. What contributes to the stability of this joint?**

The stabilizers of the glenohumeral joint can be divided into bony (static) and soft tissues (dynamic). The hard stabilizers are the **glenoid*** which is shallow and deepened by a rim of cartilage called the **glenoid labrum***. The soft stabilizers are the four muscles of the rotator cuff, i.e. **teres minor, subscapularis, supraspinatus** and **infraspinatus**; the three glenohumeral ligaments. the **superior, middle,** and **inferior glenohumeral** ligaments; the **corocohumeral ligament**; the **long head of biceps**; and the **deltoid** muscle.

22.2 Radius and ulna

> **Remember:** in anatomical terms the upper limb is divided into the arm and forearm (and the lower limb into the thigh and leg).

Typical questions

1. **Please identify this specimen and its key features**

This is a left elbow which is made up of three bones, the **humerus***, **ulna*** and **radius***, and three joints, the ulnar-humeral, the radio-humeral, and the **proximal radio-ulnar joint**.

The shaft of the humerus flares into the **capitellum*** laterally which articulates with the **radial head***. The **lateral epicondyle*** on the outside of the capitellum is the site of attachment for the **radial collateral ligament** and the common extensors of the forearm. The medial column of the distal humerus flares into the **trochlea** which articulates with the **trochlea notch*** of the proximal ulna. Medially is the **medial epicondyle*** which is the site of attachment for the **ulnar collateral ligament** and the origin of the common flexors of the forearm. Posteriorly is the **olecranon fossa*** where the olecranon rests when the elbow is in full extension.

The **trochlear notch*** is bordered by the **olecranon***, which is the site of insertion of triceps, and the **coronoid process***. Distal to the coronoid is the **ulnar tuberosity***, site of attachment of brachialis.

The proximal radius starts with the **radial head*** which articulates with the capitellum. Distal to this is the **radial neck** and **radial tuberosity***, site of insertion of the **biceps tendon.**

2. What structures might be injured in a displaced supracondylar fracture of the humerus, and how would you test these?

The brachial artery and median nerve are vulnerable in this sort of injury. They can be tested by palpating the radial and ulnar artery at the wrist, and checking sensation of the index finger and ability to form a 'O' with the tip of index finger and thumb (the 'OK' sign).

22.3 Wrist and hand

Typical questions

1. Can you identify the bones in this hand and wrist?

The eight carpal bones anticlockwise from the **radial styloid** are the **scaphoid***, **trapezium***, **trapezoid***, **capitate***, **hamate, pisiform, triquetrum***, and **lunate***.

Remember: S, T, T, C, H, P, T, L—Some Teenage Tantrums Cause Huge Problems To Lecturers.

The **metacarpals*** articulate with the distal row of carpals. The fingers have three rows of phalanges—**proximal***, **intermediate***, and **distal***. In the thumb there are just **proximal*** and **distal phalanges***.

2. What are the bony attachments of the flexor retinaculum (transverse carpal ligament)?

The flexor retinaculum is a thick fibrous sheet that lies of the volar aspect of the carpal bones forming the **carpal tunnel**. It is attached to the **scaphoid tubercle***, the **trapezium tubercle***, the **hook of the hamate***, and the **pisiform***.

3. What is the significance of the blood supply of the scaphoid to the orthopaedic surgeon?

The scaphoid bone is commonly fractured after a fall on to an outstretched hand. It is not always significantly displaced and so it may be difficult to diagnose on early radiographs. Because the nutrient vessels enter predominantly in the distal half of the scaphoid, a fracture may result in avascular necrosis of the proximal pole.

22.4 Hip joint

Typical questions

1. Please identify this specimen

This is a left hemipelvis and proximal femur including the hip joint.

2. What are the key bony features and attachments?

The **pelvic** or **innominate bone** is made up of three bones: the **ileum***, **ischium***, and **pubis***. The **anterior superior iliac spine*** is the site of attachment for **sartorius** and the **inguinal ligament**; the **anterior inferior iliac spine*** is the site of attachment for **rectus femoris** and the **iliofemoral ligament**. The **inferior*** and **superior pubic rami*** form the **obturator foramen***. The **pubic tubercle*** is the site of insertion of the **inguinal ligament*** Posteriorly, the **sacrospinous ligament** arising from the **ischial spine*** divides the **greater*** and **lesser sciatic foramen***.

The **femoral head*** articulates with the **acetabulum***. The **femoral neck*** ends at the **intertrochanteric line*** between the **greater*** and **lesser trochanters***. **Gluteus medius** and **minimus, vastus lateralis, superior gemellus,** and **obturator internus** are all attached to the greater trochanter. **Iliopsoas** inserts into the lesser trochanter.

3. Why does the leg commonly lie shortened and externally rotated following a fracture of the neck of the femur?

The action of the iliopsoas on the lesser trochanter can externally rotate and pull the femoral shaft proximally.

4. What is the blood supply of the femoral head?

The blood supply to the femoral head is from three sources. The most important is the **retinacular arteries** which run distal to proximal and are branches of the lateral and medial circumflex arteries which form an arterial anastomotic ring at the base of the femoral neck. They both arise from deep femoral artery. It is the retinacular arteries, which pierce the joint capsule before entering the femoral neck, that are disrupted during an intracapsular femoral neck fracture.

There is also a minor contribution from the **fovea artery** which lies in the **ligamentum teres** between the acetabulum and femoral head and from intramedullary branches of the **femoral nutrient arteries.**

> This is a common question because of the significance of the precarious femoral head blood supply in managing fractured femoral necks. Because displaced femoral neck fractures have a high rate of avascular necrosis they are often managed with hemiarthroplasty, especially in elderly people.

22.5 Knee

Typical questions

1. Identify this specimen, the key bony features, and the soft tissues not apparent

This is a right knee, with the distal **femur*** and proximal **tibia*** and **fibula***. The articular surface of the medial and **lateral femoral condyles*** articulates with the **tibial condyles** via the **lateral*** and **medial menisci***. Anteriorly the menisci are linked by the transverse ligament.

The **intercondylar eminence*** is the site of insertion for the two cruciate ligaments. The **anterior cruciate ligament** arises from the **lateral femoral condyle** and the **posterior cruciate** from the **medial femoral condyle***. The **popliteus** arises from the **medio-posterior tibial plateau*** and inserts into the **lateral femoral epicondyle***.

The **medial collateral ligament** runs between the **anterior-medial aspect of the tibial plateau*** and the **medial epicondyle***. The **lateral collateral ligament** runs from the **fibular head*** to the **lateral femoral epicondyle***.

Gerdy's tubercle* on the anterior-lateral tibial plateau is the site of insertion of ilio-tibial band.

The **patella*** is a sesamoid bone which is the site of insertion of the quadriceps tendon. It has two **articular facets*** that articulate with the femoral condyles. The **patellar tendon** arises from the inferior pole to insert into the **tibial tuberosity***.

2. Tell me more about the menisci

The menisci are semilunar fibrocartilage structures that lie over their respective tibial condyles. They are attached to the intercondylar eminence at each pole and on their outer edge to the joint capsule. They deepen the articular surface slightly and serve to absorb shock and spread load within the joint.

3. What is the purpose of the popliteus tendon?

In full extension, the knee joint is slightly externally rotated, which 'locks' the joint. In order to 'unlock' the joint to allow flexion, the popliteus muscle internally rotates the tibia relative to the femur.

4. What factors resist the dislocation of the patella?

The patella typically dislocates laterally because of the 'Q angle' which results in the net effect of the quadriceps muscles pulling the patella laterally. This is resisted by the **intercondylar grove***, the action of **vastus medialis**, and the **medial retinaculum.**

22.6 Foot and ankle

This is a subject which comes up in examinations with great regularity. Candidates should be aware that the standard that the examiners expect is familiarity with tendinous insertions, not just being able to name the tarsals—although candidates still attend the examination being unable to do this.

Typical questions

1. Please identify this specimen and name all of the bones

This is a left foot and ankle, comprising the **distal tibia*** and **fibula*** and the tarsal bones: **talus***, **calcaneum***, **naviculum***, **cuboid***, and **medial***, **intermediate*** and **lateral cuneiform***. There are five **metatarsals** and, analogous to the hand, the great toe has only **proximal and distal phalanges***. The other four toes have three rows of phalanges, the **proximal***, **intermediate***, and **distal phalanges***. There are two sesamoid bones under the metatarsophalangeal (MTP) joint of the great toe.

2. Which ligaments insert into the bones of the midfoot?

The calf muscles insert into the calcaneum via the **achilles tendon**, together with the **plantaris tendon**. The **tibialis posterior** inserts into the naviculum, the cuneiforms, and the 2nd, 3rd and 4th metatarsals. **Tibialis anterior** and **peroneus longus** inserts into the medial cuneiform and the base of the first metatarsal. The other **peroneal muscles** insert into the base of the 5th metatarsal.

3. What are the ligaments that stabilize the ankle joints?

There are two joints in the ankle: the distal **tibiofibular joint*** and the **mortise joint*** between the tibia, fibula, and talus. The distal tibiofibular joint is stabilized by three ligaments known collectively as the **syndesmosis**, the **anterior** and **posterior inferior tibiofibular ligaments**, and the **inferior transverse ligament.**

The ankle mortise is stabilized laterally by three ligaments: the **anterior** and **posterior talo-fibular ligaments** and the **calcaneofibular ligament**. Medially the joint is stabilized by the **deltoid ligament** which has a deep and a superficial component.

Chapter 23 **Special areas**

Some anatomical areas lend themselves very easily to viva questions and therefore occur with predictable regularity in examinations. This chapter will not provide a thorough understanding of the anatomy of these areas, but will allow candidates to convert their knowledge into punchy, accurate answers that will quickly convey both the information required and a sense of familiarity with the subject that the examiners will be looking for.

23.1 Axilla

This is relevant to both breast surgery and orthopaedics and is therefore a very common topic.

The axilla is a pyramidal intermuscular space that lies under the glenohumeral joint.

Boundaries

Apex   Lies behind middle third of clavicle

Base   Axillary fascia

Medial   Chest wall bounded by serratus anterior

Posterior • Subscapularis
              • Teres major
              • Latissimus dorsi

Lateral   • Teres major—inferiorly
              • Humerus—superiorly

Anterior   • Pectoris major
              • Pectoris minor

Contents

⤢ Brachial plexus—divisions and the three cords, named posterior, medial, and lateral in terms of their relation to axillary artery

⤢ Axillary artery—**subclavian** to **axillary** to **brachial**

⤢ Axillary vein—confluence of **basilic vein** and venae comitantes of brachial artery

⤢ Axillary lymph nodes

⤢ Axillary fat

Branches of axillary artery

Divided into three parts, relating to pectoralis minor:

⤢ 1st part (superior to pectoralis minor):
  • Superior thoracic artery

⤢ 2nd part (behind pectoralis minor):
  • Acromiothoracic artery
  • Lateral thoracic artery

⤢ 3rd part (inferior to pectoralis minor):
  • Subscapular artery
  • Anterior circumflex artery
  • Posterior circumflex humeral artery

Remember: 1st part has one branch, 2nd part has two branches, and 3rd part has three branches.

Levels of axillary lymph nodes

Divided into three groups, relating to pectoralis minor:

⤢ Level 1—inferior to pectoralis minor

⤢ Level 2—behind pectoralis minor

⤢ Level 3—superior to pectoralis minor

23.2 Upper arm compartments

The upper arm is a fascial envelope divided into two muscular compartments by the **medial and lateral intermuscular septa**, which run from the deep fascia of the arm to blend with periosteum of the humerus.

Flexor compartments

Muscles

Three muscles
- Flex elbow
- Innervated by **musculocutaneous nerve** (from lateral cord, C5–C7)

⤢ Biceps:

- Long head arises from superior glenoid
- Short head arises from coracoid with coracobrachialis via conjoined tendon
- Inserts into radial tuberosity
- Flexes elbow, supinates forearm (think of tightening screwdriver with right hand) and weakly flexes/abducts shoulder

⤢ Brachialis:

- Arises from lower half of anterior humerus and inserts into ulna tuberosity; acts as a powerful flexor of the elbow

⤢ Coracobrachialis:

- Arises from coracoid (as conjoined tendon with short head of biceps)
- Inserts into medial humerus and flexes shoulder

Neurovascular contents

⤢ Brachial artery

⤢ Median nerve

⤢ Ulnar nerve

(Radial nerve enters flexor compartment halfway down humerus via foramen in lateral intramuscular septum.)

Extensor compartments

⤢ Triceps:

- Extends elbow joint
- Innervated by radial nerve from posterior cord (C6–C8)
- Three heads—long, medial, and lateral—arising from inferior glenoid, lateral, and medial humerus respectively
- Inserts into olecranon

⤢ Proximal radial nerve

23.3 Antecubital fossa

The antecubital fossa is an intermuscular space, inverted triangular in shape, that lies on the anterior aspect of the elbow joint.

> Often introduced with a scenario of a patient with a laceration to the anterior elbow, with the candidate invited to describe the boundaries, the structures that might be transacted, and what they supply.

Boundaries

Base	Line between medial and lateral epicondyles
Medial	Lateral edge of pronator teres
Lateral	Medial edge of brachialis (overlying radial nerve)
Roof	Deep fascia of arm, (reinforced with bicipital aponeurosis) with median cubital vein overlying, not a content of the antecubital fossa
Floor	Brachialis and supinator

Contents

From medial to lateral:

↗ Median nerve

↗ Brachial artery branching into ulnar and radial arteries (and accompanying veins)

↗ Biceps tendon

↗ Radial nerve (lying under brachialis)

> **Remember:** 'NAT'—nerve, artery, and tendon.

23.4 Forearm compartments

The forearm is enveloped by deep fascia and divided into a flexor (anterior) compartment and extensor (posterior) compartment by the intermuscular septae, the radius and ulna, and the interosseous membrane.

> Remember, clinicians who deal with this area use acronyms. If you do this too in the examination situation, not only will your answers be more fluent, but you will appear more clinically experienced. Again, this topic is commonly introduced with a scenario of a patient with a laceration injury, with the candidate invited to discuss the structures likely to be injured. Knowledge of the innervation of the forearm muscles and the associated palsies is commonly examined.

Flexor compartments

↗ Divided into two groups: superficial and deep flexors

↗ All muscles innervated by median nerve *except* flexor carpi ulnaris (FCU) and flexor digitorum profundus (FDP) to little and ring fingers (ulnar two digits and ulnaris are ulnar nerve)

Superficial flexors (medial to lateral)

↗ Flexor carpi ulnaris (FCU)

↗ Palmaris longus (PL)

↗ Flexor digitorum superficialis (FDS)

↗ Flexor carpi radialis (FCR)

↗ Pronator teres (PT)

Deep flexors (medial to lateral)

↗ Flexor digitorum profundus (FDP)

↗ Flexor pollicis longus (FPL)

↗ Pronator quadratus (PQ)

Deep flexors innervated by anterior interosseous nerve, a branch of median nerve. (Except ulnar half of FDP).

Extensor compartments

Divided into superficial and deep extensors:

Superficial extensors (medial to lateral)

↗ Extensor carpi ulnaris (ECU)

↗ Extensor digiti minimi (EDM)

↗ Extensor digitorum communis (EDC)

↗ Extensor carpi radialis brevis (ECRB)

↗ Extensor carpi radialis longus (ECRL)

↗ Brachioradialis

Deep extensors (medial to lateral)

↗ Supinator

↗ Extensor indicis (EI)

↗ Extensor pollicis brevis (EPB)

↗ Extensor pollicis longus (EPL)

↗ Abductor pollicis longus (APL)

Innervated by **posterior interosseous nerve**, a branch of radial nerve.

23.5 Carpal tunnel

Space between the concavity of the **volar aspect** of the carpal bones and the **flexor retinaculum.**

Flexor retinaculum is quadrangular fibrous thickening of deep palmar fascia with corners attached to the **pisiform**, hook of **hamate, trapezium,** and **scaphoid**. Its proximal border is the distal wrist crease.

This is a very common topic in the MRCS examination, again usually introduced with the scenario of a laceration to the area and questions regarding the structures damaged and the resultant palsies.

Contents

↗ Median nerve (lies between FCR and PL)

↗ Tendons of:

• FDS (× 4)

• FDP (× 4)

• FCR

• FPL

Remember: 1 nerve and 10 tendons

Overlying the flexor retinaculum

↗ Palmaris longus

↗ Cutaneous branch of median nerve

> **Guyon's canal**
> - Separate from the carpal tunnel
> - Lies on the ulnar side of the carpal tunnel and superficial to it
> - Transmits the **ulnar nerve** and **artery**

23.6 Extensor compartments

Six extensor compartments on dorsal aspect of carpal bones, lying under the extensor retinaculum that runs between radial and ulnar styloid:

↗ I–APL, EPB

↗ II–ECRL, ECRB

↗ III–EPL

↗ IV–EDC, EI (EI lies on ulna side of EDC to index finger)

↗ V–EDM

↗ VI–ECU

23.7 Femoral triangle

The femoral triangle is an inverted triangular, gutter-shaped, intermuscular space in the upper anterior thigh.

> This is a very common examination topic, often introduced with a scenario requiring venous access in a shut-down patient. You may be asked to describe the landmarks of the femoral vein, its relations, and what might be the consequence of damaging the femoral nerve, along with more obvious questions on femoral hernias, etc.

Boundaries

Base	Inguinal ligament
Medial border	Adductor longus (lateral edge)
Lateral border	Sartorius (medial edge)
Roof	Fascia lata
Floor	• Iliacus
	• Psoas major
	• Pectineus
	• Adductor longus

Contents

The order of the femoral structures, lateral to medial, is femoral nerve, artery, and vein.

> **Remember:** NAVY—<u>N</u>erve, <u>A</u>rtery, <u>V</u>ein, and <u>Y</u>-fronts!

Femoral sheath

Extension of extraperitoneal fascia for 3 cm through femoral ring.

Consists of three compartments:

⤢ Lateral—femoral artery

⤢ Middle—femoral vein

⤢ Medial—femoral canal (node of Cloquet)

Femoral ring

Anterior border   Inguinal ligament

Medial border   Lacunar ligament

Posterior border   Pectineal ligament

Lateral border   Femoral vein

> Candidates must remember that the speciality stream of Limbs and Spine is *not* Orthopaedics. Areas like the femoral triangle that are clinically encountered in general surgery will be examined in this speciality stream, not in Trunk and Thorax.

23.8 Adductor canal

The adductor canal (also known as the canal of Hunter)is a trough-shaped intramuscular space lying in the anterior/middle aspect of the distal two-thirds of the thigh; it is a continuation of the femoral triangle.

Boundaries

Lateral border   Medial border of vastus medialis

Medial/floor   Adductor magnus and longus

Roof   Subsartorial fascia

Contents

⤢ Saphenous nerve (only structure to pass down full length of canal)

⤢ Nerve to vastus medialis

⤢ Femoral artery

⤢ Femoral vein

> Femoral artery and vein leave adductor canal halfway down its course, via the **adductor hiatus** in the **adductor magnus**, to enter the popliteal fossa where they become popliteal vessels.

23.9 Upper leg compartments

The upper leg (thigh) is divided into anterior and posterior compartments by intramuscular septum running from the **fascia lata** to the femur. The anterior compartment contains the **quadriceps muscles** and **sartorius** and the posterior compartment contains the hamstring and adductors.

Anterior compartments

⤢ Quadriceps muscle group and sartorius

⤢ Innervated by **femoral nerve** (L2–L4)

⤴ Quadriceps extend knee:
- Rectus femoris
- Vastus medialis
- Vastus intermedius
- Vastus lateralis

⤴ Sartorius flexes hip and knee

Posterior compartments

Hamstrings (semimembranosus and semitendinosus)

⤴ Sciatic nerve (L4, L5, S1–S3)

⤴ Arise from ischial tuberosity

⤴ Insert into tibia

⤴ Flex knee

Adductors

⤴ Innervated by obturator nerve (L2–L4)

⤴ Consist of
- Obturator externus
- Adductor brevis
- Adductor longus
- Adductor magnus
- Gracilis

23.10 Popliteal fossa

The popliteal fossa is a diamond shaped intramuscular space that lies behind the knee joint.

> This topic may be introduced by an examiner inviting the candidate to discuss the differential diagnosis of a popliteal swelling.

Boundaries

Upper medial	Hamstrings
Upper lateral	Biceps femoris
Lower medial	Medial head of gastrocnemius
Lower lateral	Lateral head of gastrocnemius
Roof	Popliteal fascia
Floor—above knee	Posterior femur
–behind knee	Posterior joint capsule
–below knee	• Oblique popliteal ligament • Popliteus fascia

Contents

From superficial to deep:

⤴ Sciatic nerve

⤴ Popliteal vein

↗ Popliteal artery

↗ Popliteal fat and lymphatics

↗ Bursae (closed or open, i.e. communicate with knee joint)

Remember: NirVanA : from superficial to deep = nerve, vein, artery.

23.11 Lower leg compartments

The lower leg contains four compartments bound by the **deep fascia** and separated by the tibia, fibula, interosseous membrane, anterior and posterior septae, and the **deep transverse fascia**. There are four separate muscular nerves, each of which supplies all the muscles in its compartment.

This is commonly introduced to candidates with a scenario of a patient with **compartment syndrome.**

Anterior compartment

↗ All contents pass under the extensor retinaculum to enter foot

↗ Anterior tibial artery (becomes dorsalis pedis in foot)

↗ Four extensors supplied by **deep peroneal nerve** (L4, L5, S1):

- Tibialis anterior

- Extensor hallucis longus (EHL)

- Extensor digitorum

- Peroneus tertius

Lateral compartment

↗ All contents pass behind lateral malleolus, under the lateral retinaculum, to enter foot

↗ Two everters supplied by **superficial peroneal nerve** (L5, S1):

- Peroneus longus

- Peroneus brevis

Superficial posterior compartment

↗ All contents supplied by **tibial nerve** (L5, S1, S2)

↗ Three plantar flexors that insert into calcaneum:

- Gastrocnemius

- Soleus

- Plantaris

Deep posterior compartment

↗ Muscles supplied by **tibial nerve** (L5, S1, S2)

↗ Contents pass behind medial malleolus, covered by flexor retinaculum, forming tarsal tunnel

Contents

From anterior to posterior:

↗ Tibialis posterior

↗ Flexor digitorum longus

⤢ Posterior tibial artery

⤢ Posterior tibial vein

⤢ Posterior tibial nerve

⤢ Flexor hallucis longus

Remember: 'Tom, Dick, And a Very Nervous Harry', i.e. Tibialis posterior, flexor Digitorum longus, posterior tibial Artery, posterior tibial Vein, posterior tibial Nerve and flexor Hallucis longus.

Chapter 24 **Peripheral nerves**

Peripheral nerves are an excellent examination topic; unlike 'listing the causes of …' the information is unambiguous and provides a quick way for an examiner to differentiate a well prepared candidate from a poorly prepared one. Peripheral nerve lesions are common and chronic and therefore excellent clinical exam cases, which can then lead to a mini-viva on the anatomy.

Checking sensation in a specific area is a quicker method of establishing the height of a suspected lesion than trying to remember the precise segmental dermatomal distribution. In most lesions sensation is affected before power.

A patient with a discrete nerve injury is a popular clinical scenario for examiners; preparation requires memorizing the nerve supply to the dermatomes and myotomes and practising a methodical examination technique.

24.1 Dermatomes and myotomes

	Dermatome	Myotome
Cervical		
C4	Clavicles	
C5	Deltoid tuberosity	Shoulder abductors
C6	Lateral forearm	Elbow flexors
C7	Middle finger	Elbow extensors
C8	Ulnar styloid	Ulnar deviation of wrist
Thoracic		
T1	Medial epicondyle	Finger adduction
T2	Axilla	
T4	Nipples	
T10	Umbilicus	
Lumbar		
L1	Groin	Hip flexors
L2	Anterior thigh	Hip flexors
L3	Knee	Hip adductors/knee extensors
L4	Medial malleolus	Ankle dorsiflexors
L5	Great toe	Great toe extension
Sacral		
S1	Lateral malleolus	Great toe flexion
S2	Back of knee	Great toe flexion
S5	Perianal	

See diagram of dermatomes (Fig. 24.1).

24.2 Brachial plexus

The brachial plexus is the convergence and divergence of a great number of nerve fibres running between the upper limb and spinal roots C5 to T1.

If asked about the brachial plexus in the examination, being able to draw a rudimentary line diagram whilst explaining the structure is advantageous.

See diagram of brachial plexus (Fig. 24.2).

↗ Roots (5):

- C5 to T1
- Emerge between **scalenus anterior** and **medius**
- Enter axilla by passing over 1st rib and **behind subclavian artery**

↗ Trunks (3):

- Over 1st rib in posterior triangle of neck
- Upper trunk—C5, C6
- Middle trunk—C7
- Lower trunk—C8, T1

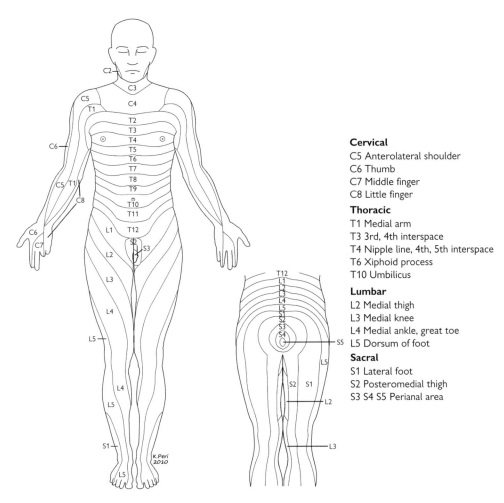

Fig. 24.1 Dermatomes.

Cervical
C5 Anterolateral shoulder
C6 Thumb
C7 Middle finger
C8 Little finger

Thoracic
T1 Medial arm
T3 3rd, 4th interspace
T4 Nipple line, 4th, 5th interspace
T6 Xiphoid process
T10 Umbilicus

Lumbar
L2 Medial thigh
L3 Medial knee
L4 Medial ankle, great toe
L5 Dorsum of foot

Sacral
S1 Lateral foot
S2 Posteromedial thigh
S3 S4 S5 Perianal area

⤢ Divisions (6):
  • Lie behind clavicles
  • Anterior (flexors) and posterior (extensors) divisions from each trunk
⤢ Cords (3):
  • Lie behind pectoralis minor
  • Posterior cord—convergence of all three posterior divisions
  • Lateral cord—convergence of anterior divisions from upper and middle trunks
  • Medial cord—anterior division of lower trunk
⤢ Major branches (5):
  • Axillary nerve from posterior cord
  • Radial nerve from posterior cord
  • Musculocutaneous nerve from lateral cord
  • Ulnar nerve from medial cord
  • Median nerve from lateral and medial cord

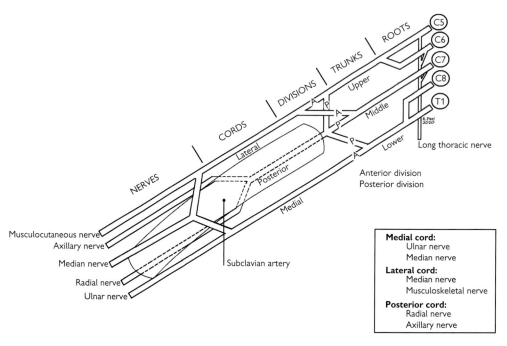

Fig 24.2 Brachial plexus.

24.3 Axillary nerve (C5, C6)

Course

↗ Arises from the posterior cord

↗ Passes through quadrangular space with posterior circumflex artery (quadrangular space delineated by both **teres** muscles and long and **lateral heads of triceps** and humerus)

↗ Circles around surgical neck of humerus

Supplies

↗ Motor:

• Deltoid

• Teres minor

↗ Sensory:

• Skin over deltoid 'regimental badge' area

Test

↗ Motor:

• Shoulder abduction

↗ Sensory:

• Regimental badge area

Vulnerable areas: injured in anterior glenohumeral dislocation or fractures of proximal humerus.

24.4 Musculocutaneous nerve (C5–C7)

Course

- ⤢ Arises as the continuation of lateral cord
- ⤢ Pierces **corocobrachialis** and passes toward elbow between **biceps** and **brachialis**
- ⤢ Below elbow, pierces deep fascia of forearm to continue as lateral cutaneous nerve (sensory only) of forearm

Supplies

- ⤢ Motor:
  - Muscles of anterior compartment of the upper arm:
    - Biceps brachii
    - Brachialis
    - Corocobrachialis
- ⤢ Sensory:
  - Lateral surface of forearm

Test

- ⤢ Motor:
  - Elbow flexion
- ⤢ Sensory:
  - Lateral surface of forearm

Vulnerable areas: rarely injured in proximal humeral fractures.

24.5 Ulnar nerve (C7, C8, T1)

Course

- ⤢ Arises from medial cord of brachial plexus
- ⤢ Runs medial to brachial artery in upper arm, and pierces intermuscular septum (via **arcade of Struthers**) to lie on anterior of triceps
- ⤢ Passes behind medial epicondyle (cubital tunnel) at elbow
- ⤢ Runs deep to muscle of FCU, then radial to its tendon
- ⤢ Lies on ulnar side of ulnar artery as both structures pass through **Guyon's canal**

Supplies

- ⤢ Motor:
  - FCU
  - FDP to little and ring fingers
  - Adductor pollicis
  - Four hypothenar muscles:
    - Palmaris brevis
    - Abductor digiti minimi (ADM)
    - Flexor digiti minimi (FDM)
    - Opponens digiti minimi (ODM)

- All interosseous muscles
- 3rd and 4th lumbricals

↗ Sensory:

- Ulnar half of hand, little finger, and half of ring finger

Tests

↗ Motor:

- Froment's test—thumb **adduction** against a piece of paper
- Crossing fingers
- Finger **abduction** against resistance

↗ Sensory:

- Pulp of little finger

> Vulnerable area: cubital tunnel syndrome and Guyon's canal. Remember the ulnar paradox, that a more proximal ulnar nerve lesion produces a less pronounced 'ulnar claw' since the FDP is also paralysed.

24.6 Median nerve (C6–C8, T1)

> A very common examination topic because of the high incidence of carpal tunnel syndrome and median nerve injury at the wrist.

Course

↗ Arises from **medial** and **lateral cords** of brachial plexus

↗ Travels down medial aspect of upper arm, crossing superficial to brachial artery midway down upper arm

↗ Enters forearm between heads of **pronator teres**

↗ Gives off **anterior interosseous nerve** in proximal forearm (supplying FDP to index and middle, FPL, and pronator quadratus)

↗ Gives of palmar cutaneous branch just before carpal tunnel

↗ Median nerve then passes under flexor retinaculum

Supplies

↗ Motor:

- All flexor muscles of forearm except FCU and FDP to little and ring fingers
- Three of four thenar muscles:
  - Abductor pollicis brevis (APB)
  - Opponens pollicis (OP)
  - Flexor pollicis brevis (FPB)
  - 1st and 2nd lumbricals

↗ Sensory:

- Radial aspect of palm
- Palmar aspect and nail bed of index, middle, and radial half of ring finger

Tests

↗ Motor

- Ability to **abduct** thumb against resistance while palpating thenar eminence

↗ Sensory:

- Sensation at pulp of index

Vulnerable areas: cubital fossa in lacerations or supracondylar humerus fractures and carpal tunnel due to lacerations, distal radius fractures, or carpal tunnel syndrome.

24.7 Radial nerve (C6–C8, T1)

Course

↗ Arises from posterior cord

↗ Leaves axilla and passes through **triangular space** (between long head of triceps, teres major and humerus)

↗ Runs down **spiral groove** of posterior humerus, before crossing into anterior/flexor compartment between brachioradialis and brachialis

↗ Passes anterior to lateral epicondyle and branches into superficial (cutaneous) and deep nerves

↗ The deep branch becomes **posterior interosseous nerve** after piercing supinator (supplying muscles of extensor component of forearm except ECRL whose branch is given off before division)

Supplies

↗ Motor:

- Arm:
  - Triceps, anconeus, brachioradialis
- Forearm:
  - All extensors, supinator, and APL

↗ Sensory:

- Posterior aspects of arm and forearm
- Dorsal aspect of thumb, and dorsal index, middle and half ring, excluding nail beds

Tests

↗ Motor:

- Extension of wrist/fingers against resistance

↗ Sensory:

- Sensation in 1st web space dorsally

Vulnerable areas: **axilla/triangular space** in 'crutch palsy', midshaft humerus fracture, and radial head fracture.

24.8 Upper limb palsies

Erb–Duchenne's

↗ C5 and C6 upper brachial plexus injury from a fall with shoulder/neck abducted (in adults), or a traction on head in childbirth

↗ Results in 'waiter's tip' position, i.e. an inability to abduct shoulder or flex elbow, arm hanging by trunk, palm backwards

Klumpke's claw-hand

↗ T1 lower brachial plexus injury

↗ Usually caused by traction on arm in childbirth

↗ Appearance due to paralysis of **lumbricals** which normally flex metacarpophalangeal joint (MCPJ) and extend IPJs

Radial nerve palsy

↗ Inability to extend elbow, supinate forearm, extend wrist and fingers, depending on level

↗ Classically causes wrist drop due to pressure on radial nerve as it passes adjacent to humeral shaft—**crutch or Saturday night palsy**

Ulnar nerve palsy

↗ Often due to injuries at elbow/wrist (look for fracture deformities)

↗ Also caused by longstanding pressure behind medial epicondyle (cubital tunnel syndrome)

↗ Results in palsy of ring and little fingers with wasting of interosseous muscles, most visible in 1st web space

Median nerve palsy

↗ Often due to elbow/wrist penetrating trauma

↗ Loss of forearm pronation and wrist flexion if injured at wrist

↗ Wasting of thenar eminence

↗ Loss of abduction of thumb

↗ Palsy affecting only thenar muscles most commonly due to longstanding carpal tunnel syndrome

24.9 Lumbar plexus

The lumbar plexus is a condensation of nerve fibres from the **anterior rami of L1–L4** and lies within the substance of psoas major.

↗ Branches:

↗ Femoral (L2–L4)

↗ Obturator (L2–L4)

↗ Also:

- Iliohypogastric
- Ilioinguinal
- Genitofemoral

24.10 Femoral nerve

Course

↗ Arises from L2–L4 via lumbar plexus

↗ Travels deep to belly of psoas major to emerge and pass under inguinal ligament just lateral to femoral artery in femoral sheath

↗ Branches 2–3 cm inferior to inguinal ligament

↗ Gives off saphenous nerve—only part of femoral nerve which descends below knee, sensory only

Supplies

↗ Motor:

- Anterior thigh muscles:
  - Quadriceps
  - Pectineus
  - Sartorius

↗ Sensory:

- Contributes to joint sensation of hip and knee
- Anterior and lower medial thigh, via medial and intermediate cutaneous nerves of thigh
- Medial lower leg and foot

Tests

↗ Motor:

- Extension of knee

↗ Sensory:

- Lower medial thigh

24.11 Obturator nerve

Course

↗ Arises from L2–L4 via lumbar plexus

↗ Descends in belly of psoas major, before emerging medially at the level of pelvic brim and descending behind common iliac vessels

↗ Gives off no branches before leaving pelvis via obturator foramen

Supplies

↗ Motor:

- Obturator externus
- Adductor magnus
- Adductor brevis
- Adductor longus

↗ Sensory:

- Upper medial thigh
- Hip and knee joint

Tests

↗ Motor:

- Hip adduction

↗ Sensory:

- Upper medial thigh

Vulnerable areas: obturator hernia can compress nerve.

24.12 Sciatic nerve (L4, L5, S1–S3)

The lumbrosacral plexus is a condensation of the **anterior rami of the sacral nerve roots S1–S3 and** a contribution from L4 and L5. It principally gives rise to the **sciatic nerve**, the thickest nerve in the body. The sciatic nerve supplies the posterior compartment of the thigh and, via its terminal branches, almost everything below the knee. The posterior cutaneous nerve of thigh, which comes off the plexus, supplies the posterior aspect of the thigh as far as the popliteal fossa with sensation.

Course

- ↗ Arises from L4, L5, S1–S3 via lumbrosacral plexus
- ↗ Leaves pelvis via the greater sciatic foramen below piriformis
- ↗ Passes exactly halfway between ischial tuberosity and greater trochanter
- ↗ Travels down thigh between hamstrings and adductor magnus
- ↗ Gives off branches to some posterior compartment muscles
- ↗ Just superior to popliteal fossa, branches into **common peroneal** and **tibial nerves**

Supplies

- ↗ Motor:
  - Semitendinosus
  - Semimembranosus
  - Biceps femoris
  - Adductor magnus (with obturator nerve)

Tests

- ↗ Motor:
  - Flexion of the knee
- ↗ Sensory:
  - Sciatic nerve not sensory above knee

Vulnerable areas: damaged in posterior dislocation of hip, during hip replacement, or by penetrating injury (e.g. buttock IM injections).

24.13 Tibial nerve (L4, L5, S1–S3)

The tibial nerve (Fig. 24.3) is larger than the peroneal (fibular) nerve and supplies the superficial and deep posterior compartments of the lower leg.

Course

- ↗ Arises by the branching of the sciatic nerve, a variable point just above the upper border of the popliteal fossa
- ↗ Lies in the **popliteal fossa**, superficial to the vein and artery
- ↗ Passes behind medial malleolus before branching into **medial** and **lateral plantar nerves**

Supplies

- ↗ Motor:
  - Gastrocnemius
  - Soleus
  - Plantaris

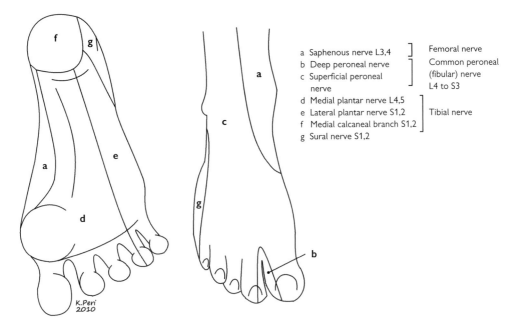

a Saphenous nerve L3,4 ⎤ Femoral nerve
b Deep peroneal nerve ⎤ Common peroneal
c Superficial peroneal ⎥ (fibular) nerve
  nerve ⎦ L4 to S3
d Medial plantar nerve L4,5 ⎤
e Lateral plantar nerve S1,2 ⎥ Tibial nerve
f Medial calcaneal branch S1,2 ⎥
g Sural nerve S1,2 ⎦

Fig 24.3 Sensory supply of the foot.

- Deep compartment:
  - Tibialis posterior
  - Flexor digitorum longus
  - Flexor hallucis longus
- ⬀ Sensory:
  - Knee joint
  - Lateral leg, foot, and 5th toe
  - Sole of the foot

Tests

⬀ Motor:
- Plantarflexion

⬀ Sensory:
- Sole of foot

24.14 Peroneal (fibular) nerve (L4, L5, S1, S2)

This smaller of the two terminal branches of sciatic nerve supplies the anterior and lateral compartment of the lower leg. It is increasingly referred to as the common fibular nerve, especially by anatomists; however, for the examination, the term 'peroneal' is probably less likely to confuse.

Course

⬀ Runs along medial boarder of biceps femoris in popliteal fossa

⬀ Passes round fibular neck

⬀ Enters lateral compartment and branches into deep and superficial peroneal nerves

Supplies

⤢ Superficial peroneal nerve:
  - Lateral compartment:
    - Peroneus longus
    - Peroneus brevis
    - Dorsal foot sensation
⤢ Deep peroneal nerve:
  - Anterior compartment:
    - Tibialis anterior
    - EDL
    - EHL
    - Peroneus tertius
    - 1st web space sensation

Tests

⤢ Motor:
  - Extension of great toe
⤢ Sensory:
  - Dorsum of foot

> Vulnerable areas: very commonly injured, as common peroneal nerve passes around fibular neck either by direct trauma or by chronic pressure from an over-tight below-knee cast.

Chapter 25 **Limb vasculature**

This is an area that may clinically lie in the realm of vascular surgery, not orthopaedics. The candidate may be tempted to regard limbs and spine as being the 'orthopaedic theme' and although that is largely true, there should be no doubt that not only do all candidates need a knowledge of this area, but it may well be examined in a specified limbs and spine station.

25.1 Upper limb arteries

The arterial supply of the upper limb is from the axillary/brachial artery and its two terminal branches: the radial and ulnar arteries.

Axillary artery

Divided into three parts by the overlying pectoralis minor.

Each part gives off a corresponding number of branches:

↗ 1st part:
- Above pectoralis minor
- Superior thoracic artery

↗ 2nd part:
- Underlying pectoralis minor
- Thoracoacromial artery
- Lateral thoracic artery

↗ 3rd part:
- Below pectoralis minor
- Subscapular
- Anterior circumflex artery
- Posterior circumflex artery

> Classic examination question: remember the parts of the axillary artery are numbered in the opposite direction to the levels of axillary lymph nodes.

Brachial artery

↗ Continuation of axillary artery distal to axilla

↗ Axillary artery runs down upper arm deep to biceps brachii, adjacent to median nerve

↗ Passes through antecubital fossa between median nerve and biceps tendon

↗ Divides into **radial** and **ulnar arteries** over the neck of the radius

> **Remember: Allen's test** for determining the relative contribution of the radial and ulna arteries to the blood supply of the hand. Both arteries are excluded with direct pressure, the fist is clenched to exsanguinate the hand and then either the radial or ulnar arteries is released, then the test is repeated with the other artery tested. The speed of reperfusion is compared to determine the dominant artery.

25.2 Upper limb veins

The veins of the upper limb are more complicated and prone to more variation than those of the lower limb. Like the arterial supply, venous drainage of the upper limb depends ultimately on a principal vessel, the **axillary vein**. The axillary vein is the confluence of **the basilic and cephalic veins.**

Cephalic vein

⤢ Originates just dorsal to the radial styloid at the wrist

⤢ Gives off a branch to basilic vein, the median cubital vein

⤢ Lies very superficial at the antecubital fossa—a key point for venepuncture

⤢ Ascends upper arm in grove between brachioradialis and biceps

⤢ Pierces deep fascia and lies under deltoid

⤢ Joins axillary vein just below clavicle

Basilic vein

⤢ Lies in the forearm just anterior to the superficial ulnar border

⤢ Communicates with the cephalic vein via the median cubital vein

⤢ Pierces deep fascia midway up upper arm

⤢ Joins with the venae comitantes of the axillary arteries to form the axillary vein

> This topic has been introduced in the examination by asking candidates to identify sites for emergency venous access on a cadaveric specimen.

25.3 Lower limb arteries

Femoral artery

⤢ Continuation of the external iliac artery below the inguinal ligament at the midinguinal point (halfway between anterior superior iliac spine and pubic symphysis

⤢ Immediately gives off **superficial epigastric artery** (key landmark in inguinal hernia repair)

⤢ 5 cm below inguinal ligament, gives off **profunda femoris artery**

⤢ Profunda femoris gives off the **medial** and **lateral circumflex femoral arteries** which supply the hip joint and the four perforator arteries of the thigh

⤢ Femoral artery proper passes through **adductor canal (of Hunter)**

⤢ Femoral artery becomes the popliteal artery in the popliteal fossa

> Clinically this is a very significant area within surgery and therefore a very common examination topic. It has been examined both by cadaveric specimens with arteries labelled with flags, and by angiogram images.

Popliteal artery

⤢ Continuation of the femoral artery below the adductor hiatus (in **adductor magnus**)

⤢ Divides into its three terminal branches of anterior and posterior tibial arteries and peroneal (or fibula) artery

Anterior tibial artery

⤢ Pierces the interosseous membrane and lies in the anterior compartment

⤢ Passes under extensor retinaculum between the EHL and tibialis anterior

⤢ Palpable as dorsalis pedis before it passes between the 1st and 2nd metatarsals

Posterior tibial artery

⤢ Passes deep to soleus, in the midline of the lower leg in the deep posterior compartment

⤢ Gives off perforators 5, 10, and 15 cm above medial malleolus

⤢ Passes under flexor retinaculum **between posterior tibial vein** and **nerve** where it is palpable

Peroneal artery

↗ Runs in deep posterior compartment and gives off penetrating arteries 5 cm and 10 cm above lateral malleolus

> The perforating branches of the posterior tibial and peroneal arteries which arise at predictable heights, and at **5 cm intervals**, from the **medial and lateral malleoli** respectively, are vulnerable during a fasciotomy.

25.4 Lower limb veins

Questions regarding the superficial veins of the lower limb are likely to be the mainstay of the examination, as these have surgical relevance both as grafts for vascular and cardiac surgery, and as pathological varicose veins. The deep veins accompany their partnered arteries; the superficial veins are long and short saphenous veins.

Long saphenous vein

↗ Passes 2 cm anterior to medial malleolus

↗ Reliably lies 4 cm posterior to the medial edge of patella

↗ 2.5 cm below inguinal ligament, the long saphenous vein pierces deep fascia to join the femoral vein, medial to palpable femoral artery

Short saphenous vein

↗ Lies behind the lateral malleolus

↗ Pierces deep fasica over politeal fossa and joins popliteal vein

> The site of the long saphenous vein in relation to the medial malleolus is a common examination topic, often introduced with the scenario of an injured patient who needs a venous cut-down.

Section 2 Pathology and Physiology

Chapter 26 **Fractures**

This topic is easily introduced in the exam with a radiograph showing a fracture. When formulating your answer, **always** consider the whole patient and make reference to the Advanced Trauma Life Support (ATLS™) principles. For example:

'I would approach this patient according to the ATLS™ protocols and once I had established that there were no life-threatening injuries I would assess the fracture....'

26.1 Describing fractures

It is likely that if you are asked to describe a fracture, it will be of a common and simple type, e.g. distal radius or neck of femur. Avoid jumping straight to eponymous names, but describe the fracture using technical terms and only offer eponymous names or classification systems if you are very confident of your knowledge.

If it is a special case, i.e. neck of femur or ankle, describe it in special terms. For example,

'This a mortise view of a right ankle showing a bimalleolar fracture of the distal tibia and fibula'

or

'This is an AP view of the pelvis showing an intracapsular fracture of the left femoral neck.'

Site

↗ Describe the radiograph (briefly), including patient's name and rough age (do not waste time calculating exact age if it is not clear immediately)

↗ Name the fractured bone, including the side, if clear from the radiograph

↗ Describe the position of the fracture, i.e. distal, proximal, midshaft, etc.

Orientation

↗ State whether there are only two fragments or multiple fragments, i.e. a **simple** fracture or a **multifragmentary** fracture

↗ Describe the orientation of the fracture line—**transverse**, **oblique** or **spiral**

↗ State if the fracture crosses an articular surface, i.e. **intra-** or **extra-articular**

Displacement

↗ How much have the two fracture fragments separated or moved? In other words, is the fracture **undisplaced** or **minimally displaced**?

↗ Describe the displacement in terms of percentage displacement of the two fracture surfaces, or if there is no contact, 'off-ended'

Angulation

↗ Describe the direction and degree of the angulation of the **distal** fragment. For example,

'This is an AP film of the right wrist showing a fracture of the distal radius. The fracture is transverse, extra-articular, minimally displaced but dorsally angulated.'

If asked what further information you would like to ascertain, that is normally a prompt to consider the neurovascular status of the limb or the soft tissues around the fracture: i.e. is it an open injury?

26.2 Fracture management

This is unlikely to be a main focus of an examination station, but may form the basis of one or two final questions. Always avoid leaping to an immediate answer; rather, take the examiner through the possible options, demonstrating your knowledge before opting for a specific technique. Remember the principles: reduce fracture, hold reduction until healed, and rehabilitate.

Conservative/nonsurgical

↗ Do nothing, e.g. undisplaced radial head fractures

↗ Splintage, e.g. plaster cast

↗ Traction, either skeletal or skin

Surgical

↗ Reduction and insertion of Kirschner (K) wires

↗ External fixation, e.g. pelvic fractures

↗ Extramedullary: **open reduction and internal fixation (ORIF)** with plates and screws

↗ Intramedullary(IM): IM nail

↗ Arthroplasty

↗ Excision

26.3 Fracture healing

Fractured bone can heal in two ways: direct or indirect.

Direct healing

↗ Also called **primary fracture healing**

↗ Occurs when the fracture is anatomically reduced and absolutely stable

↗ Occurs with ORIF with screws and plates

↗ Does not involve callus formation

↗ Relies on haversian remodelling with osteons crossing the fracture (provided gap <1 mm) absorbing necrotic bone and laying down new bone tissue

Indirect healing

↗ Also called **secondary fracture healing**

↗ Occurs when there is **relative** not **absolute** reduction and stable fixation, i.e. fracture approximation

↗ Occurs with splintage, external fixation, or IM nailing

↗ Involves five phases:

- Haematoma phase: 0–48 hours
  - ≋ Haemorrhage forms haematoma in and around fracture gap
  - ≋ Fibrin mesh becomes matrix for inflow of inflammatory cells
- Inflammatory phase: 2–7 days
  - ≋ Neutrophils and macrophages migrate into haematoma, releasing cytokines activating osteoprogenitor cells and fibroblasts.
- Soft callus: 1–3 weeks
  - ≋ Chondroblasts replace fibrin mesh with collagen, stabilizing fracture
- Hard callus: 3–12 weeks
  - ≋ Endochondral ossification occurs as bone replaces cartilage
- Remodelling: 3+ months
  - ≋ Disordered new bone undergoes remodelling as woven type bone is replaced by lamellar bone

26.4 Complizations of fractures

Complications of disease, injuries or surgery is a very common question. It should always be approached systematically, for example:

'I will divide the complications into local and general and into immediate, early, and late.'

Immediate

- ↗ Associated injuries i.e. polytrauma, brain injury, neurovascular or muscle damage
- ↗ Haemorrhage

Early

- ↗ General acute respiratory distress syndrome (ARDS), fat emboli, pneumonia
- ↗ Deep venous thrombosis/pulmonary embolism (DVT/PE)
- ↗ Local wound infection, **compartment syndrome**

Late

- ↗ Malunion (healing in unsatisfactory position)
- ↗ Nonunion (hypertrophic or atrophic)
- ↗ Avascular necrosis (e.g. femoral head and scaphoid)
- ↗ Osteoarthritis, in intra-articular fractures
- ↗ Complex regional pain syndrome

Compartment syndrome is such an important fracture complication that it is often the subject of follow-up questions. It occurs when there is 'a rise in pressure in a myofascial compartment'. It is primarily a clinical diagnosis which warrants immediate surgical decompression, i.e. fasciotomy. It is characterized by 'pain out of proportion to the injury despite analgesia, exacerbated by passive stretching of muscles within the compartment'. Invasive compartment pressure measurement is diagnostic if there is < 30 mmHg pressure difference between compartmental and diastolic pressures.

26.5 Factors that affect bone healing

Local

- ↗ Infection
- ↗ Excessive movement
- ↗ Inadequate reduction
- ↗ Inadequate blood supply (often due in part to excessive soft tissue dissection during operative fracture management)

General

- ↗ Comorbidities, e.g. diabetes
- ↗ Drugs, e.g. steroids and NSAIDs
- ↗ Smoking
- ↗ Poor nutrition

Section 3 **Clinical**

Chapter 27 **Common cases**

As has previously been mentioned, it is in the three clinical stations—one history based, and two physical examinations—that the real bias towards the chosen specialities manifests. If you have chosen Limbs and Spine as your speciality, your history station and one of your two physical examination stations will be in this area.

27.1 Dupuytren's contracture

The chronic nature of this condition, and its painlessness in examination, makes it a very popular choice for the examiners to present to a candidate. Almost certainly it will be in a physical examination rather than a history station.

> Candidates still attend the MRCS examination believing that Dupuytren's contracture involves the flexor tendons. An answer like that will vex the examiners!

Examination

Inspect	• Age, sex, and ethnicity of patient
	• Affected hand (if allowed ask about hand dominance and profession)
	• Affected digits
Palpate	Feel to confirm which digits and/or whether the palm is affected
Move	Move each of the relevant joints in the digit and remember the range of movement (RoM)

Present

'This is a middle-aged, right-handed man with a Dupuytren's contracture. He has a contraction cord affecting his left ring finger palmar fascia. His RoM at the MCPJ is limited to 50–90° but unaffected at the proximal and distal interphalangeal joints (PIPJ/DIPJ).'

Likely questions

1. What patient factors are associated with Dupuytren's?

↗ Diabetes mellitus

↗ Alcohol intake

↗ Sex (M:F 4:1)

↗ Family history

↗ Northern European ethnicity

2. What is the underlying pathology?

The exact pathophysiology is unknown, but there is hyperplasia of the longitudinal myofibroblasts in the palmar and digital fascia.

3. What are the management options?

The management options are either surgical or conservative. Surgery is indicated if the contracture causes functional implications, e.g. unable to place hand in pocket, poking eyes when washing face, etc. Surgery involves a Z-plasty and then excision of the contracture bands. The condition will reoccur in about 25% of cases. If the contracture is longstanding, there may not be recovery of a full RoM.

27.2 Rheumatoid hand

This is a very common case for a physical examination station. Be aware that the patient might be tender by the end of the OSCE session, so be gentle. With all 'hand' cases, expose both of the patient's upper limbs to above the elbow. The appearance of the rheumatoid hand is classical and the 'look' part of the physical examination is most important: count to 10 slowly in your head as you gently turn the patient's hands over, and flex their elbows to inspect their ulnar borders, and thus convincing the examiner of your meticulous and considered approach to the case.

Examination

Inspect
- Age and sex of the patient
- Swelling of MCPJ
- Spindling of fingers
- Ulnar deviation of fingers at MCPJ
- Radial deviation at the wrist
- Rheumatoid nodules along ulna, toward elbow
- 'Swan-neck' deformity of DIPJ
- 'Boutonniere' deformity of PIPJ
- Scars near the joints

Palpate Gently feel all joints of hand of wrist for swelling

Move
- Check elbow, forearm and wrist movements
- Check grips—power, tripod, key, and precision ('squeeze my fingers, pick up this pen, hold this key, pick up this coin')

Present

'This is a middle-aged woman with a symmetrical polyarthritis affecting the small joints of her hands. There is swelling of her MCPJs with ulnar deviation of her fingers. There is a swan-neck deformity of all fingers and rheumatoid nodules at both elbows. I note the well-healed, longitudinal, dorsal scar over the right wrist, which, together with the lack of movement of this joint, likely represents a wrist arthrodesis (fusion). There is a functional limitation with difficulties of all grips apart from power grip. I believe this patient has rheumatoid arthritis.'

Likely questions

1. How can you clinically differentiate between rheumatoid arthritis and osteoarthritis?

Rheumatoid arthritis (RhA) is an inflammatory disease of the synovial membrane of joints and tendon sheaths. Osteoarthritis (OA) is a degenerative condition articular surface of the joints. RhA affects mainly the MCPJs and the wrist which are swollen, while OA affects mainly the DIPJs and thumb carpal–metacarpal joint (CMCJ) which have nodules. Severe deformity caused by joint subluxation, and nodules, are seen only in RhA.

2. What is the structural abnormality underlying swan-neck and boutonniere deformities?

These deformities, characteristic of RhA, are caused by the destruction of the extensor mechanism and unbalanced action of the intrinsic muscles.

3. What are the surgical options for treating RhA of the hand?

The mainstay of management of RhA is medical with anti-inflammatories and disease-modifying agents. However, surgical options include synovectomy or arthrodesis of the wrist joint and MCPJ arthroplasty.

27.3 Osteoarthritic hand

This is less common than a RhA case in the examination, as the signs are less florid. The classic appearance of the OA hand is described as the 'square hand', due to OA degeneration of the thumb carpometacarpal (CMC) joint causing subluxation.

Examination

Inspect
- Age, sex, and ethnicity of patient
- Affected hand (if appropriate, ask about hand dominance and profession)
- Heberden's and Bouchard's nodes—osteophytes at DIPJ and PIPJs respectively
- Thumb CMCJ subluxation and prominence

Palpate	Osteophytes at DIPJ (Heberden's nodes) and PIPJ (Bouchard's nodes)
Move	Check RoM in fingers—extension normally preserved with limited extension
Test	'Grind test' of thumb CMC (mention to examiner without performing, as it is painful)

Heberden's nodes are most prominent and are osteophytes at base of distal phalanges.

Present

'This is a right-handed, middle-aged woman who has the appearance of degenerative changes affecting her right thumb CMCJ. Prominent Heberden's nodes are visible at the DIPJ and palpable Bouchard's nodes at the PIPJ. Gross movement is preserved, but power is reduced. She has osteoarthritis affecting the joints of her hand.'

Likely questions

1. How would you manage this patient's condition?

Management options in this case are conservative and surgical. Conservative options include nonsteroidal anti-inflammatory analgesia, physiotherapy, and splintage. Surgical options are limited. If thumb CMCJ symptoms predominate, then the trapezium can be excised. Arthoplasty or arthrodesis of the other joints of the hand has a very limited role.

2. What are the classic changes of osteoarthritis visible on plain radiograph?

Loss of joint space, subchondral sclerosis, subchondral cysts, and osteophytes.

27.4 Osteoarthritis of the knee or hip

This case can be introduced as either OA or as a post arthroplasty. It is also a common case for a history station.

Examination

Inspect	• Age
	• Walking stick
	• Evidence of tibial plateau of distal femur fracture/surgery
	• Muscle wasting
	• Arthroplasty scars—midline for knees, lateral–posterior for hips
	• Knee/hip held in slight flexion relative to contralateral limb
	• Varus (more common) or valgus deformity
Feel	• (Hip) palpate groin and over greater trochanter and ask which corresponds to pain
	• (Knee) warm, prominent ostephytes
Move	• Loss of RoM especially internal rotation in hip
	• Loss of flexion and extension in knee and feel for patella crepitus during movement

Present

'This middle aged man, who appears to use a walking stick, is holding his right knee in a semi-flexed position. His knee appears swollen and has a varus deformity. The right knee is slightly warmer than the left and has a RoM of 10–80° with marked crepitus on movement. He has advanced osteoarthritis in his right knee.'

Likely questions

1. How would you investigate this patient and what findings would you expect?

After a full history and examination I would request an AP and lateral plain radiographs. I would expect to see the radiological signs of OA, i.e. a loss of joint space with greater loss in the medial joint in this case, subchondral sclerosis, and cysts and osteophytes.

2. What are the management options for this patient?

The management options can be divided into conservative or surgical. Conservative include physiotherapy, behaviour modification, analgesia, and intra-articular steroid injection. The surgical option is arthroplasty. For early changes in the knee of a young patient, osteotomy has an occasional role.

History points

The diagnosis of major joint OA is usually fairly obvious: it is a progressive, chronic condition that may worsen throughout the day or after inactivity. The principle aim of the history is to rule out differential diagnosis and elucidate the impact and severity of the condition.

* ⤢ Differential diagnosis OA knee: meniscal tear, cruciate rupture, occasionally RhA
* ⤢ Differential diagnosis OA hip: RhA, avascular necrosis, septic arthritis, hernia (femoral/inguinal), sequelae of congenital dysplasic hip, metastases, or impacted fracture

Ask about:

* ⤢ Night sweats—septic arthritis, especially TB
* ⤢ Trauma—fracture, meniscal tear or cruciate rupture
* ⤢ Weight loss/history of cancer—metastases
* ⤢ Childhood hip problems or operation—developmental dysplasia of the hip
* ⤢ Surgery—arthroplasty or knee arthroscopy

27.5 Ganglion

A chronic, relatively painless condition that lends itself well to examinations.

Examination

Inspect	• Age and hand dominance • Lump, usually around the wrist, subcutaneous
Palpate	• Cystic, uniform, fluctuant tethered to deep structures, may be able to reduce volume of ganglion with pressure • May be quite tender
Move	May move with excursion of tendons around the wrist

Present

'This right-handed woman in her thirties has a smooth uniform lump on the dorsal aspect of her right wrist. It is nonpulsatile, deep to the skin, cystic, and tethered to deep structures. This is a ganglion.'

Likely questions

1. What is a ganglion?

A ganglion is a herniation of the synovial membrane forming a cyst which contains synovial fluid.

2. What are the treatment options?

The treatment options are divided into either intervention or conservative. Intervention involves either aspiration or excision under a regional or general anaesthetic. The reoccurrence/resolution rate at 5 years is about the same with either excision or no intervention.

3. What are the risks of excision?

Reoccurrence rate of approximately 20% over 5 years, infection, painful scar, vascular damage and bleeding, and damage to nerves and tendons with loss of function in the hand. Anaesthetic risks.

27.6 Trigger finger

The chronicity and close relationship between disease and anatomy make this a favourite in examinations.

Examination

Inspect • Age, sex, and hand dominance
 • Isolated of flexion of middle or ring finger
 • Possible signs of other associated conditions (e.g. diabetes, gout, RhA)
 • Patient may extend the affected finger with the other hand

Palpate Tender nodule in the flexor tendon sheath, just below A1 pulley

Move Finger can be fully extended with a 'click'.

Present

'This man in his sixties is holding his ring finger in isolated flexion. There are no signs of contracture cords. There is a slightly tender nodule in the ring finger flexor sheath. The finger can be eased into extension, and after this, there is a normal range of movement. This patient has a trigger middle finger.'

Likely questions

1. What is the anatomical basis of this condition?

Normally a minor injury or overuse results in a nodule of inflammation within the FDS tendon that gets stuck as it passes under the A1 pulley.

2. How would you distinguish between this and Dupuytren's disease?

In Dupuytren's, there is a fixed flexion deformity and presence of cords in the palmar fascia. In trigger finger, full extension can normally be achieved and the palmar fascia is normal.

3. What are the treatment options for trigger finger?

The management options are conservative or operative. Conservative options include NSAIDs and steroid injection into the flexor sheath. The A1 pulley can be surgically divided but this is rarely necessary as steroid injections are normally effective.

27.7 Ulnar nerve palsy

This is a question that leads very easily to questions on the supply of the ulnar nerve. Chronic ulnar deficits are relatively common from trauma or untreated compression syndromes.

Examination

Inspect • Age, sex, dominance
 • Obvious abnormal hand position, i.e. claw hand
 • Scarring around wrist or elbow from either surgery or trauma
 • Deformity at elbow indicating previous fracture
 • Interosseous muscle wasting in the hand

Palpate Test for sensation at little finger pulp, index finger pulp, and first web space

Move • Hold the elbow and check movement, feeling for obvious abnormal movement indicative of previous trauma
 • Check power in hand muscles: **abduction** of index/little finger against resistance, ability to cross fingers

Tests **Card test—adduction** of index finger (palmar interossei) by patient resisting you pulling a card from between their index and middle finger

 Froment's test of thumb adduction (adductor policis) by patient resisting you pulling a card held between extended thumbs and index finger, when palms opposed

 Tinel's test at superficial sites of nerve compression, i.e. Guyon's canal and cubital tunnel

Present

'This is a middle-aged, right-handed man. He is holding his left hand in the position of an 'ulnar claw', with his left ring and little finger extended at the MCPJ and flexed at the interphalangeal joint (IPJ). There is muscle wasting of the 1st web space. Sensation is reduced in the ulnar nerve distribution, but otherwise normal. Finger abduction is weak and the card test and Froment's test are positive for weakness in the ulnar-supplied muscles. Tinel's test at the cubital tunnel causes pain in the little and ring fingers. This patient has cubital tunnel syndrome, causing compression of his left ulnar nerve.'

Likely questions

1. Explain the appearance of the ulnar claw hand in terms of anatomy of the muscles involved and their nerve supply

The ulnar nerve supplies the lumbricals in the little and ring fingers. The lumbricals act to flex the MCPJ and when they are denervated, the action of the extensors on the MCPJ is unopposed. Although the FDP to these fingers is also lost, with a high ulnar nerve lesion the FDS acts to flex the PIPJ, creating a claw-like appearance.

2. What is meant by the term 'ulnar paradox'?

If the lesion of the ulnar nerve is at the wrist, then the FDP to the little and ring finger is preserved and therefore both of the IPJs are flexed which, with the hyperextended MCPJs, make the deformity appears more pronounced than a higher lesion which involves loss of FDP action.

3. What are common causes of an ulnar nerve lesion?

The common causes of ulnar nerve damage from proximal to distal are: penetrating injury at the axilla, a distal humeral fracture, compression in cubital tunnel syndrome, and penetrating trauma at the wrist or compression in ulnar tunnel syndrome.

27.8 Median nerve palsy

This is a very common case in the examination, because patients with median nerve palsy from untreated carpal tunnel syndrome are so common.

> Remember that although a median nerve palsy might have resulted from carpal tunnel syndrome, this syndrome is often classically intermittent in nature. Carpal tunnel syndrome is likely to be introduced by the examiner with a description such as 'this patient attends clinic complaining of intermittent paraesthesia in her fingers'.

Examination

Inspect
- Age, sex, and hand dominance
- Wasting of thenar eminence
- Wrist deformity indicating previous distal radius fracture
- Scars over carpal tunnel indicating trauma or previous surgery
- Evidence of conditions associated with carpal tunnel syndrome: RhA, pregnancy, DM, obesity, hypothyroidism

> Symptoms of carpal tunnel syndrome occur in order of pain ('pins and needles'), numbness, and finally weakness. Once weakness occurs, decompression is unlikely to reverse it, only to remove pain.

Palpate Test sensation in medial nerve distribution: palmar aspect of thumb, index and middle finger; exclusively to index pulp

Move Test power in abductor pollicis (exclusively supplied by median nerve)

Tests
  • **Phalen's test**—aggravation of symptoms of pain and numbness when wrist flexed for 30–60 seconds

  • **Tinel's test**—tapping firmly over the carpal tunnel reproduces symptoms

> The median nerve is said to supply sensation to the palmar aspect of thumb, index, and middle fingers, and power to the LOAF muscles: <u>L</u>umbricals (radial two), <u>O</u>pponens pollicis, <u>A</u>bductor pollicis, <u>F</u>lexor pollicis brevis. However, because of mixed supply with the ulnar nerve, exclusive median supply is only to sensation in the index finger and power to abductor pollicis.

Present

'This woman in her sixties reportedly suffers from shooting pain in her right thumb and index and middle fingers. On examination there are no scars but dorsal angulation of the wrist. She has wasting of her right thenar eminence and reduced sensation in her median distribution. Thumb abduction is very weak. Neither Tinel's or Phalen's test worsens her symptoms. I believe she has median nerve compression at the carpal tunnel, possibly secondary to a distal radius fracture.'

Likely questions

1. If the patient has carpal tunnel syndrome, would Tinel's and Phalen's test be negative?

If the carpal tunnel syndrome was chronic, as is suggested by the presence of muscle weakness and wasting, then early symptoms of pain might have been replaced by numbness and Phalen's and Tinel's tests would be unlikely to exacerbate their symptoms.

2. Do you know other tests for carpal tunnel syndrome?

The gold standard test is nerve conduction studies, but an additional bedside test is the tourniquet test where a tourniquet is inflated on the arm to occlude arterial flow, exacerbating symptoms.

3. What are the treatment options for carpal tunnel syndrome?

If carpal tunnel syndrome is likely to be secondary to a reversible or temporary cause such as pregnancy or hypothyroidism, this can be addressed. Steroid injections into the carpal tunnel and splintage are sometimes used, but the main treatment is surgical decompression which can be performed under local or regional anaesthetic.

4. What specific risks would you warn a patient about carpal tunnel decompression under local anaesthetic?

Recurrence or failure to fully resolve symptoms, damage to nerves or tendons with loss of function in the hand, infection, wound breakdown, and a chronic painful scar. The palmar sensory and recurrent motor branches can be damaged.

27.9 Radial nerve palsy

This is the least likely of the upper limb nerve palsies to occur in the examination, because it is the least common clinically, and is anatomically simpler.

Examination

Inspect
  • Age, sex, and hand dominance
  • 'Wrist drop', i.e. wrist resting in flexed position
  • Scars of surgery or trauma at humerus and elbow

Palpate
  Test sensation at 1st web space dorsally

Move
  Test elbow extension and wrist extension

> The Medical Research Council (MRC) grading of muscle power is from 5 to 1. Grade 5 is normal power, 4 is active movement against gravity but weaker than 'normal', 3 is active movement against gravity, 2 is active movement with gravity excluded, 1 is a flicker of action and 0 is no contraction.

Present

'This middle-aged, left-handed man has an apparent right-sided wrist drop at rest. There are no signs of trauma or surgery. Sensation is reduced in the 1st web space and although elbow extension against resistance is powerful, wrist extension is weak. I think this man has a right radial nerve lesion, possible at the level of the distal arm or elbow.'

Likely questions

1. What are the causes and sites of radial nerve lesion?

Penetrating trauma can damage the nerve at almost any site. The radial nerve at the axilla is vulnerable to pressure, for example in 'crutch palsy'. In the arm, the radial nerve is also vulnerable to pressure in 'Saturday night palsy' or humerus fracture or surgical fixation. Dislocation of the elbow, or fractures around it, can damage the nerve. The nerve can also become compressed in the supinator muscle.

27.10 Diabetic foot

Examination

Inspect	• Age and sex • Signs of cigarette smoking • Ulcers, hairless legs • Missing toes (autoamputation or surgical) • Neuropathic arthropathy
Palpate	• Temperature difference between feet • All pulses bilaterally from groin to dorsalis pedis and tibialis posterior • Capillary refill at toes • Sensory loss in stocking distribution
Move	Proprioception in toes

Present

'This woman in her sixties has signs consistent with smoking. In her right foot there is an ulcer under her heel and deformity of her 1st metatarsophalangeal joint (MTPJ). She has reduced sensation in both feet in a stocking distribution, but with loss to a higher level on the right. All leg pulses are present bilaterally but capillary refill is prolonged to 5 seconds in the toes on the right. There is a loss of proprioception in the great toes on the right. This patient has a signs of peripheral neuropathy with a heel ulcer and arthropathy of her 1st MTPJ. The most likely underlying cause is diabetes.'

Likely questions

1. What investigations would you order?

If this was a new presentation I would investigate the likely underlying diabetes with a fasting glucose and an HbA_{1c} assay. With specific regard to the foot I would request plain radiographs of the foot to look for possible osteomyelitis of the heel and to determine the extent of destruction in the 1st MTPJ.

2. How should this patient's condition be managed?

This patient should be managed by a multidisciplinary team with efforts to optimize glycaemic control and smoking cessation being central. Foot care should involve a podiatrist and will most likely involve an air-cushioned protective boot.

3. What is the scope for vascular surgery in this case?

The presence of peripheral pulses but prolonged capillary refill suggests microvascular disease rather that major vessel disease that might be amenable to surgical treatment.

27.11 Varicose veins

Cases of 'barn door' varicose veins may well also show more subtle signs of venous insufficiency, which is a more important diagnosis to make.

Examination

Inspect
- Age and sex
- Engorged, tortuous veins
- Superficial thread vein
- Oedema
- Venous ulcers
- Signs of stasis dermatitis including haemosiderin deposition, eczema, and lipo-dermatosclerosis

Palpate
- Palpate veins to determine how high they start
- Check to see if oedema is pitting

Test
Tredelenburg's test to determine the competence of the valves between the deep and superficial veins

Present

'This middle-aged man has obvious varicose veins affecting his right leg. They are most prominent around the calf and there are no signs of them above the knee. There is pitting oedema and mild discoloration of haemosiderin around the ankle. There is an area of erythema just proximal to the medial malleolus, but the skin has not broken down. Trendelenburg's test indicates that there is valvular incompetence below the knee. The diagnosis is varicose veins caused by venous insufficiency.'

Likely questions

1. What one investigation would you be most interested in to confirm this diagnosis?

Venous Doppler ultrasound scan: this will confirm the valvular incompetence indicated by the clinical examination and localize it precisely.

2. Tell me about the communicating veins between the deep and superficial venous systems

There are communicating veins between the short saphenous vein and the deep veins 5, 10 and 15 cm above the medial malleolus.

3. What is the likely treatment in this case?

The oedema and haemosiderin deposition indicate that the deep venous system may be deficient and therefore stripping of the superficial varicose veins would be contraindicated. The mainstay of treatment in this case is therefore likely to be graded compression stockings.

Chapter 28 **Special tests**

Knowledge of the right special tests to use in a given case is how you let the examiner know that you are not just automatically performing the examination but are thinking about the findings as you go along and have chosen an appropriate way to differentiate between diagnoses, or gain more information about a diagnosis. In short, it is how you show the examiner you are at the required standard to be admitted into the Royal College.

Remember: look, feel, move, special tests

This is not a detailed explanation of how to perform each and every orthopaedic special test, rather when to use them, what you are testing, and what the results mean.

It is sometimes challenging to remember if a test is positive if abnormal or normal. In the examination, rather than trying to remember, explain the results as you understand them: for example:

'Froment's test indicated a right-sided weakness of adductor pollicus consistent with an ulnar nerve lesion.'

28.1 Froment's test

Tests	For power of adductor pollicis and therefore its innervation by the ulnar nerve
Used	When you suspect an upper limb nerve deficit (NB you must also check ulnar sensation)
Performed	By asking patient to place their hands palm to palm, then asking them to grip a piece of paper placed between their index fingers and thumbs **while keeping their thumbs straight**. If, as you pull on the paper, the patient flexes one of their thumbs to resist you, this implies that adductor pollicis is weak as they are compensating with FPL, which is innervated by the median nerve

28.2 Card test

Tests	For power of the palmar interosseous muscles and therefore their innervation by the ulna nerve
Used	When you suspect an upper limb nerve deficit (NB you must also check ulnar sensation)
Performed	By placing a piece of paper between their extended index and middle finger and asking patient to resist your pulling the paper away. Compare sides to determine relative weakness (NB you must also check ulnar sensation)

28.3 Phalen's test

Tests	For carpal tunnel syndrome by provoking symptoms
Used	If a patient reports intermittent median nerve compression symptoms
Performed	By maximally flexing both wrists for 30–60 seconds to provoke symptoms (NB not very sensitive or specific). Reverse Phalen's with wrists maximally extended can be performed in addition

Remember: Phalen's flexing, Tinel's tapping.

28.4 Tinel's test (sign)

Tests	For nerve irritation by provoking symptoms
Used	Typically when history suggests carpal or ulnar nerve syndrome
Performed	By firmly (perhaps less firmly in the examination) percussing (with index and middle fingers) over suspected area of nerve compression/irritation, e.g. carpal or cubital tunnel

28.5 'Empty can' test

Tests	Power of supraspinatus muscle
Used	When patient gives a history of shoulder pain
Performed	By fully extending elbow, extending shoulder to 90°, and abducting to 20–30°. The arms are then internally rotated as if emptying out the contents of a can. The patient is then asked to resist gentle downward pressure on the elbow

28.6 Finkelstein's test

Tests	For De Quervain's tenosynovitis by provoking the symptoms
Used	When patient's give a history of wrist pain, especially around the radial aspect

Performed By gripping the patient's thumb and using it to quickly ulnar deviate the patient's wrist, provoking symptoms

28.7 Grip tests

Tests   Hand function

Used   In cases with hand deformity or other cause of function loss, e.g. RhA

Performed By asking patient to demonstrate each type of grip in turn using props:
- Power/palmar grip—ball
- Hook grip—plastic bag
- Tripod grip—pen
- Tip pinch grip—pin
- Pulp pinch—coin
- Lateral pinch—key

You are unlikely to be expected to examine grips in a station. But in a RhA hand case, you may well be asked about different types of grip.

28.8 Straight leg raise

Tests   For sciatic nerve irritation by a prolapsed disc by provoking symptoms

Used   With history of leg pain associated with lumbar symptoms

Performed By lying patient flat on their back, and lifting their straight leg off the couch to the point when the patient is in pain. To be true sciatic symptoms, the pain /paraesthesia must be felt below the knee

28.9 Trendelenburg's sign

Tests   The power of gluteus medius and minimis (hip abductors) or most commonly their pain inhibition due to hip OA

Used   For assessment of hip, following history of pain

Performed By asking patient to stand on affected leg for 30 seconds. Normally the contralateral side of pelvis rises as the ipsilateral iliac wing is pulled down by the hip abductors. If the abductors are not strong enough to do this, the contralateral side dips

28.10 Trendelenburg's test

Tests   The competence of the valves between deep and superficial veins in the legs

Used   To determine the level of incompetent valves in a patient with varicose veins

Performed By lying patient on their back, and raising their leg to drain the veins of blood. A blood-pressure cuff is then inflated and the patient stood up. Valves are regarded to be incompetent if superficial veins refill in less than 35 seconds

Trendelenburg was a German surgeon who trained in Scotland. His eponymous test and sign are often (wrongly) spoken of as if they were synonymous! If asked about the 'test' in an orthopaedic case, don't correct the examiner, use the correct one for the context.

28.11 Patrick's test

Tests	Arthropathy of the hip or sacroiliac joint by provoking the symptoms
Used	When a patient complains of hip pain, is thought to be positive in early OA
Performed	Placing the foot on the affected side of the supine patient on their contralateral knee and push the knee of the affected side toward the bed, forcing the hip into external rotation, provoking the symptoms

Patrick's test is also known as the FABER test because of the position of the affected limb: Flexion, Abduction, External Rotation.

28.12 Valgus/varus stress tests

Tests	The competence of the medial and lateral collateral ligaments
Used	When a patient reports knee instability or previous knee injury
Performed	By stressing the knee in a valgus and varus position with the knee fully extended then flexed 20°. Comparison should be made with uninjured side. Pain indicates sprain, while 'opening up' of knee indicates complete rupture ± cruciate rupture

28.13 Anterior draw test

Tests	For competence of the anterior cruciate ligament
Used	When a patient reports knee instability or previous knee injury
Performed	On a supine patient with knee flexed to 80°, the lower leg is firmly pulled forward, the extent of anterior draw is compared with the contralateral side

Lachmann's test relies on detecting the same abnormal displacement of tibial plateau on femoral condyles but with the knee flexed to 20° to relax the capsule and the bones held in the examiner's hands.

28.14 Posterior draw test

Tests	Posterior cruciate competence
Used	When a patient reports knee instability or previous **high-energy** knee injury
Performed	On a supine patient with knee flexed to 80°, the lower leg is firmly pushed backwards, the extent of posterior draw is compared with the other side

28.15 McMurray's test

Tests	For medial meniscal lesions
Used	When a patient reports symptoms of internal knee derangement
Performed	By fully flexing the knee, externally rotating the ankle and extending the knee with a valgus stress on the knee. A meniscal tear is revealed with a 'clunk'

Rather than performing McMurray's test in the examination, tell the examiner that you would normally do so and ask if you should proceed. It is unlikely you will be asked to do so, as it can be unpleasant for the patient, but don't rely on this!

28.16 Berger's test

Tests For arterial insufficiency in the legs

Used If such a diagnosis is suspected from the history of lack of peripheral pulses

Performed With the patient supine, the patient's legs are elevated for 45 seconds. An arterial diseased leg will go very pale, and rather than just returning to a normal pink colour upon return to the bed, it will become bright red

PART 3
HEAD AND NECK

Section 1 **Anatomy**

Chapter 29 **Pituitary anatomy**

Examination questions on the pituitary gland are common because they are an easy way to link anatomical structure to function. They are typically introduced with a cross-sectional scan or prosected head.

29.1 Overview

The pituitary gland (**hypophysis cerebri**) is both an endocrine and exocrine gland (like the adrenals, pancreas, and testis). It is 1.2–1.5 cm in diameter, occupies approximately 80% of the **pituitary fossa** (sella turcica) in which it sits, and is covered by **diaphragm sella** (a fold of dura mater pierced by the infundibulum).

Structure

- Two lobes connected by narrow zone 'pars intermedia'
- Anterior lobe is larger than posterior lobe
- Posterior lobe connected to the tuber cinereum in the floor of the 3rd ventricle via pituitary stalk (infundibulum)

> Make sure that you can locate the pituitary gland on a prosected specimen in the MRCS examination. You may also have to locate it on an MRI or CT scan.

Relations

Anterior	Tuberculum sellae and anterior clinoid processes (wing-like projections of the sphenoid bone)
Posterior	Posterior clinoid process
Inferior	Sphenoid body
Lateral	Cavernous sinuses and contents
Superior	Optic chiasm (immediately in front of the infundibulum)

> **Remember:** this close relationship to the optic chiasm and the unyielding nature of the other relations explain the mass effect of a pituitary tumour.

29.2 Posterior pituitary

The posterior pituitary is also called the neural lobe or **neurohypophysis**. It is embryologically and anatomically continuous with the hypothalamus, which in the basal part of the forebrain surrounding the third ventricle.

Neurons from the hypothalamus project directly to the posterior pituitary in the hypophyseal nerve tract, and hormones are released from the posterior pituitary in direct response to potentials travelling down these axons:

- Oxytocin—regulator of labour and lactation
- Antidiuretic hormone (ADH)—also known as **vasopressin**, it is a potent vasoconstrictor and also opens aquaprin water channels in collecting ducts in kidneys, promoting water retention

29.3 Anterior pituitary

The anterior lobe (adenohypophysis) is anatomically distinct from the hypothalamus and consists of a collection of endocrine cells.

Anterior lobe cells can be classified by their specific secretory products:

Somatotrophs	Somatotropin (GH)
Lactotrophs	Prolactin (PRL)
Corticotrophs	Adrenocorticotropic hormone (ACTH)

| **Gonadotrophs** | Luteinizing hormone (LH) and follicle stimulating hormone (FSH) |
| **Thyrotrophs** | Thyroid stimulating hormone (TSH) |

> The posterior pituitary produces **oxytocin** and **ADH**. The anterior pituitary produces **GH, ACTH, TSH, PRL, FSH, LH, MSH,** in response to the hypothalamic production of releasing hormones: **GHRH, ACRH, TRH, PRLRH, GnRH, POMC.**

The anterior pituitary is functionally but not anatomically connected with the hypothalamus.

Nerve cells in the hypothalamus secrete neurohormones that, via a system of hypophyseal portal vessels in the median eminence, act on the endocrine cells of the anterior lobe to stimulate or inhibit their synthesis and secretion.

29.4 Blood supply

> Be prepared to describe the blood supply of the pituitary in a viva answer, linking this to pituitary function.

The pituitary has anatomical and functional connections with the brain but sits **outside the blood–brain barrier.**

Anterior pituitary

- Receives blood supply from hypothalamic portal system
- This allows transport of releasing hormones from hypothalamus directly to anterior pituitary

Posterior pituitary

Together with the pituitary stalk, receives blood from two hypophyseal vessels:

- The **inferior hypophyseal artery** divides into branches which anastomose around the posterior lobe
- The **superior hypophyseal arteries** have anterior and posterior branches which pass into the pituitary stalk

Venous drainage

- Anterior lobe drains into the anterior hypophyseal veins
- Posterior lobe drains into posterior hypophyseal veins
- Hypophyseal veins both drain into the internal jugular vein (IJV) and therefore carry pituitary hormones into the general circulation

Chapter 30 **Thyroid and parathyroid**

30.1 Thyroid anatomy

The thyroid is an **endocrine** gland weighing 10–15 g, situated in the throat below the larynx. It consists of multiple small sacks called **follicles**. The inside of the follicle contains a viscous fluid called **colloid**, which contains mostly **thyroglobulin**, the precursor of thyroxine.

Structure

The thyroid is a butterfly shaped gland composed of:

Isthmus	Lying over the 2nd and 3rd tracheal rings
Lateral lobes	From each side of the thyroid cartilage downwards to the 6th tracheal ring
Pyramidal lobe	• Projecting upwards from the isthmus, usually on the left, representing a remnant of the thyroid's embryological descent
	• Not always present

Relations

Prosected specimens of the neck are a common way to examine candidates on thyroid anatomy. Specifically, examiners are looking for knowledge of the relations to the gland, because of their relevance in thyroid and neck surgery.

Anteriorly	• Enclosed in **pretracheal fascia**
	• Covered by strap muscles
	• Overlapped by sternocleidomastoid muscles (SCMs)
	• **Anterior jugular veins** (right and left) lie over the isthmus
	• Pretracheal fascia form thyroid capsule which is denser anteriorly—therefore large goitres extend posterior-inferiorly into superior **mediastinum**
Superiorly	• Pretracheal fascia blends with larynx, therefore thyroid moves up and down with swallowing
	• Thyroid enlargement causes the strap muscles to stretch and adhere to the gland, so that they may appear to be thin layers of fascia at operation
Posteriorly	• Larynx and trachea, with the oesophagus posterior to the trachea
	• External branch of superior laryngeal nerve (supplying cricothyroid)
Laterally	• Carotid sheaths (carotid artery, vagus nerve, IJV)
	• Recurrent laryngeal nerve (RLN) lies in groove between trachea and oesophagus

Arterial supply

⤢ Three arteries:

- Superior thyroid artery arises from the external carotid artery (ECA) and passes to the upper pole
- Inferior thyroid artery arises from the **thyrocervical trunk** of the 1st part of the **subclavian artery** and passes behind carotid sheath to posterior of gland
- Thyroid ima artery inconsistent, arises from aortic arch/brachiocephalic trunk

⤢ Also numerous smaller vessels to thyroid from trachea and pharynx

Arterial supply and venous drainage of the thyroid is a common question: it is important because awareness of the vessels is essential to prevent their injury during surgery.

Venous drainage

⤢ Superior thyroid vein—drains upper pole to IJV

⤢ Middle thyroid vein—drains lateral gland to IJV

⤢ Inferior thyroid vein—often several, drain lower pole to brachiocephalic veins

30.2 Parathyroid anatomy

Typically there are four parathyroid glands, but the number varies from two to six. Each gland is the size of a split pea, and yellow or brown. 90% lie close to the thyroid while 10% are aberrant (usually inferior) parathyroids.

Superior parathyroid

Usually lies at the middle of the posterior border of the thyroid, above the level at which the inferior thyroid artery crosses the RLN.

Inferior parathyroid

Below the inferior artery near to the lower pole of the thyroid.

Aberrant inferior parathyroids

May lie in front of the trachea after descending along inferior thyroid veins, or track further inferiorly into the superior mediastinum with thymic tissues.

Less commonly the inferior parathyroid may lie behind the fascial sheath, behind the oesophagus or in the posterior mediastinum.

Chapter 31 **Salivary glands**

31.1 Overview

Salivary function

- ↗ Keep buccal/labial mucous membrane moist
- ↗ Lubrication during mastication
- ↗ Initiate starch digestion
- ↗ Allow taste
- ↗ Prevent tooth decay

> The salivary glands and ducts can become inflamed, infected, or blocked with stones and tumours, and are injured during surgery. This ensures their clinical significance. Their complicated anatomy, which is more 'relative' than absolute, makes them a frequent topic, as it allows examiners to distinguish well-prepared candidates easily.

31.2 Parotid gland

- ↗ Largest of three salivary glands
- ↗ Produces serous saliva
- ↗ Enclosed in parotid sheath: tough fascial membrane

Location

- ↗ Located between ramus of the mandible and styloid process of the temporal bone
- ↗ Anteroinferior to external acoustic meatus and TMJ
- ↗ Apex posterior to angle of mandible
- ↗ Inferiorly overflows the mandible and overlying masseter
- ↗ Lateral surface flat and subcutaneous
- ↗ Muscles of mastication anteriorly
- ↗ Mastoid process and SCM posteriorly
- ↗ Pierces buccinator muscle.

Relations

Structures within parotid gland, from superficial to deep:

- ↗ Facial nerve and its branches
- ↗ Retromandibular (posterior facial) vein (from junction of superficial temporal and maxillary)
- ↗ ECA
- ↗ Parotid lymph nodes

> The branches of the **facial nerve (CN VII)** pass through the parotid gland, and are therefore at risk of damage during parotid gland surgery. The facial nerve branches in the parotid may form a complex network of connections. No branches emerge from the superficial aspect, which can therefore be completely exposed without risk of nerve damage.

A malignant tumour of the parotid gland may involve CN VII and produce a facial nerve palsy.

Duct

- Parotid duct (of **Stenson**) is 5 cm long
- Passes horizontally from the gland's anterior edge
- At anterior border of masseter it turns medially and pierces buccinators
- Then enters oral cavity opposite **2nd maxillary molar**

> **Sialography**: injection of radio-opaque dye into glandular duct system via duct orifice, followed by radiography. This imaging will demonstrate parts of the gland that have been displaced or dilated by disease, e.g. tumour or intraductal calculus.

Nerves

- **Auriculotemporal nerve** (branch of CN V3) is closely related to the parotid gland, passing superiorly to it with the superificial temporal vessels (sensory)
- **Great auricular nerve** (C2 and C3, a branch of the cervical plexus) innervates the parotid sheath (sensory)
- Parasympathetic part of **glossopharyngeal nerve** CN IX (via auriculotemporal nerve from the otic ganglion) supplies parotid secretory fibres
- Sympathetic nerves from **cervical nerve plexus** on ECA

Arterial supply

- Branches of ECA
- Superficial temporal artery

Venous drainage

- Retromandibular veins

Lymph drainage

- Parotid lymph nodes receive drainage from the forehead, lateral eyelids, temples, lateral auricle, external acoustic meatus, and middle ear

31.3 Submandibular gland

- Medium-sizes gland (half the size of parotid)
- Produces mixed serous and mucous saliva
- Made up of a large superficial and small deep lobe that connect around the posterior border of the mylohyoid
- Enclosed in capsule of deep fascia

Location

- Superficial lobe palpable between body of mandible and mylohyoid muscle (overlapping digastrics)
- Both superficial and deep to mylohyoid
- Hyoglossus lies deep to the submandibular gland (separated by fascial sheath), as do the lingual and hypoglossal nerves
- Superficially covered by platysma

Relations

⬈ Submandibular lymph nodes lie either side of gland, partly embedded and between it and inferior border of mandible

⬈ Lingual nerve passes inferior to duct

⬈ Facial artery approaches posteriorly, arches over superiorly (along groove), to reach the inferior border of masseter then ascends on to the face

⬈ Lies immediately lateral to **submandibular duct**

⬈ Lingual nerve to the tongue 'double-crosses' the gland

Duct

⬈ Submandibular (**Wharton's**) duct is 5 cm long

⬈ Arises from deep gland lying between **mylohyoid** and **hypoglossus**

⬈ Runs forwards beneath the floor of the mouth's mucosa (parallel to the tongue)

⬈ Opens by 1–3 orifices beside the base of the **lingual frenulum** on to an elevation (**submandibular papilla**)

Nerves

⬈ Presynaptic parasympathetic motor fibres are conveyed by the facial, chorda tympani, and lingual nerves to synapse in the **submandibular ganglion**

⬈ Postsynaptic fibres travel along arterial supply with vasoconstrictive fibres from the superior cervical ganglion

Arterial supply

⬈ Submental artery

Venous drainage

⬈ Submental veins

Lymph drainage

⬈ To deep cervical lymph nodes (especially into **jugulo-omohyoid node**)

31.4 Sublingual gland

⬈ Almond shaped, smallest, deepest salivary gland that produces mainly mucous saliva

Location

⬈ Floor of the mouth between the mandible and **genioglossus**

⬈ Separated from base of the tongue by the submandibular duct and the lingual nerve

⬈ Bilateral glands merge to form horseshoe around lingual frenulum

⬈ Lies immediately in front of deep part of submandibular gland

Ducts

⬈ Numerous sublingual glands from a series of ducts which open into the buccal floor along sublingual folds

Arterial supply

⬈ Sublingual and submental arteries (branches of facial and lingual arteries)

Nerves

Accompany nerves for submandibular gland, i.e. presynaptic parasympathetic motor fibres are conveyed by the facial, chorda tympani, and lingual nerves to synapse in the **submandibular ganglion.**

Excision of submandibular gland due to ductal calculus or tumour is not uncommon. The skin incision is made at least 2.5 cm inferior to the angle of mandible to avoid the **mandibular branch** of the **facial nerve (CN VII).**

Chapter 32 **Vascular anatomy**

This is one of the most common 'pure anatomy' areas that is the subject of questions in the MRCS examination. It is commonly introduced via a prosected specimen either in an anatomy station with key vessels flagged, or using cross-sectional imaging.

32.1 Common carotid arteries

Left common carotid artery (LCCA)

↗ Arises from **aortic arch** in front and to the right of the origin of the left **subclavian artery**

↗ Passes behind left sternoclavicular joint first in front of, then to the left of the trachea

↗ Lies medially to left lung, pleura, and phrenic nerve

Right common carotid artery (RCCA)

↗ Arises from the bifurcation of the **brachiocephalic artery** behind the left sternoclavicular joint

Both common carotid arteries (CCAs) have similar courses and relationships in the neck, ascending in the **carotid fascial sheath** which also contains the IJV laterally and vagus nerve between and deep to the artery and vein.

Relations to carotid sheath

Posteriorly	Cervical sympathetic chain
Deep	Cervical transverse processes separated by the prevertebral muscles
Medially	Larynx, trachea with the RLN, pharynx, oesophagus and thyroid gland (slightly overlapping)
Superficially	SCM and strap muscles over lower part and crossed by the intermediate tendon of omohyoid

No side branches but **bifurcates at the level of the upper thyroid cartilage (C4 level)** into the internal and external carotids (Fig 32.1).

Ligation of the common carotid artery can be performed for intracranial aneurysm arising on the internal carotid artery (ICA). This reduces the blood flow through the aneurysm, allowing thrombosis to occur. The brain on the affected side is supplied by free communication between the branches of the ECA on each side via the circle of Willis (see below)

The common carotid artery can be exposed via a transverse incision over the origin of the SCM immediately above the sternoclavicular joint. The carotid sheath lies deep to the junction between the sternal and clavicular heads of the SCM, and so can be revealed by splitting its heads or moving it laterally. Opening the sheath shows **CCA lying medial to IJV.**

32.2 External carotid artery

Initially lies deep to the anterior border of SCM, then superficial in the anterior triangle of the neck where it is visible and palpable.

Course

↗ Initially deep to carotid then passes anteriorly and laterally

↗ Lies medially to the IJV then passes anteriorly

↗ Ascends beneath **CN XII (hypoglossal nerve)** and posterior belly of digastrics to enter the parotid, where it lies **deep to CN VII (facial nerve)** and retromandibular vein

↗ Ends within parotid at the neck of the mandible by dividing into the superficial temporal and internal maxillary arteries

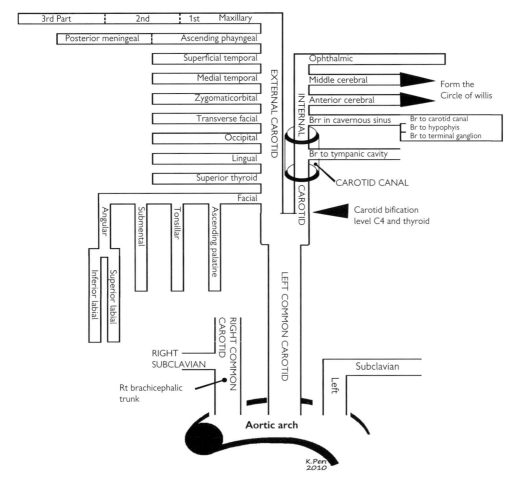

Fig 32.1 Branches of the carotid arteries.

Branches

Six branches:

⤢ Superior thyroid artery

⤢ Lingual artery

⤢ Facial artery

⤢ Occipital artery

⤢ Posterior auricular artery

⤢ Ascending pharyngeal artery

Which branches are palpable?

Facial artery over the mandible and occipital artery, over nuchal line of skull and superficial temporal artery over the **zygomatic arch.**

Terminal branches
- ↗ Superficial temporal artery
- ↗ Internal maxillary artery (IMA)
- ↗ Gives off middle meningeal *artery* (MMA)

> **MMA** is a branch of the internal maxillary artery. It lies under the weakest point in the skull, an H-shaped suture known as the **pterion**, the meeting point of the sphenoid, frontal, parietal, and temporal bones of the skull. A blow/fall on the pterion may damage the middle meningeal artery and cause an extradural haemorrhage.

32.3 Subclavian arteries

Left subclavian artery
- ↗ Arises from the **arch of the aorta** immediately posterior to the start of LCCA
- ↗ Ascends against the medial left lung and pleura (laterally), with trachea and oesophagus medially to lie deep to the left **sternoclavicular** joint

> Subclavian arterial aneurysm never involves its 1st thoracic part, usually its 3rd part. It may cause pain, weakness, and numbness because of its proximity to the brachial plexus.

Right subclavian artery
- ↗ Formed behind the right **stenoclavicular** joint by bifurcation of the **brachiocephalic artery**

Variations in subclavian origins
- ↗ Right subclavian artery may arise directly from **aortic arch** either as its 1st or last branch. If it arises as its last branch, it passes behind the trachea and oesophagus to reach the neck, and may compress the oesophagus, causing dysphagia (dysphagia lusoria)
- ↗ Left subclavian may share a common origin with the LCCA from the **aortic arch**

> A cervical rib may elevate the subclavian artery causing it to appear as an aneurysm. It may also cause vascular changes in the arm due to peripheral emboli thrown off that form on the walls of the compressed subclavian artery, and reduced blood supply to the arm

Course
The cervical course of both subclavian arteries is divided by the **scalenus anterior muscle** into three parts:
- ↗ 1st part:
  - Arches over the apex of the lung, then lies deep to SCM and strap muscles
  - Is crossed by the carotid sheath and by the **phrenic** and **vagus nerves**
  - On the right: the vagus gives off its **recurrent laryngeal** branch which hooks behind the artery
  - On the left: the thoracic duct crosses the artery to open into the left brachiocephalic vein
- ↗ 2nd part:
  - Lies deep to **scalenus anterior** which separates it from the subclavian vein
  - Lies superficial to **scalenus medius** and also middle and upper trunks of the **brachial plexus**
- ↗ 3rd part:
  - Extends to the lateral border of the first rib against which it is compressed to feel its pulse
  - Immediately deep is the **lower brachial plexus trunk**

Blalock's operation for tetralogy of Fallot: the right subclavian artery is grafted end to end to short-circuit the pulmonary stenosis.

Branches

↗ 1st part:
- Vertebral artery
- Thyrocervical trunk
- Inferior thyroid artery
- Transverse cervical artery
- Suprascapular artery
- Internal thoracic artery

↗ 2nd part:
- Costocervical trunk
- Deep cervical artery
- Superior intercostal branch
- 1st and 2nd intercostal arteries

↗ 3rd part:
- No constant branch

32.4 Internal jugular vein

The IJV runs from its origin at the **jugular foramen** (where it drains the **sigmoid sinus**).

Course

↗ Terminates behind the sternal extremity of the clavicle (joins **subclavian vein** to form **brachiocephalic vein**)

↗ First lies lateral to ICA then to CCA within the **carotid sheath**

↗ Lies next to deep cervical chain of lymph nodes (may become adherent with these nodes if malignancy/inflammation, e.g. TB)

Tributaries

↗ Pharyngeal venous plexus

↗ Common facial vein

↗ Lingual vein

↗ Superior and middle thyroid veins

32.5 Superficial veins

Superficial temporal and **maxillary veins** join to form the retromandibular vein

Retromandibular vein

↗ Branches as it crosses the parotid

↗ Its posterior division joins with the posterior auricular vein to form EJV

↗ Anterior division joins the **facial vein** to form the **common facial vein** which opens into IJV

External jugular vein (EJV)

↗ Crosses SCM in the superficial fascia

↗ Transverses the roof of the **posterior triangle**

↗ Then descends through the deep fascia 2.5 cm superior to the clavicle to enter the **subclavian vein**

↗ More easily seen with Valsava manoeuvre

↗ Occasionally double

Anterior jugular vein (AJV)

↗ Runs down either side of the neck midline, crossing the thyroid isthmus

↗ Just above the sternum both sides join, then passes outwards, deep to **SCM** to enter **EJV**

32.6 Subclavian vein

This is the continuation of the axillary vein from its commencement at the outer border of the 1st rib.

Course

↗ Crosses and slightly grooves the superior aspect of the first rib

↗ Lies behind clavicle and subclavian muscle

↗ Extends to medial border of **scalenus anterior** where it joins IJV to form the brachiocephalic vein

↗ Left subclavian vein receives the **thoracic duct**

↗ Terminates behind the sternoclavicular joint

Central line insertion

To measure central venous pressure and provide central access, e.g. for inotropic support. This is ideally carried out with ultrasound guidance.

IJV

Direct puncture in the triangular gap between the sternal and clavicular heads of SCM, immediately above the clavicle. The needle is inserted near the apex of this triangle at a 30–40° angle, whilst the carotid is palpated/ultrasound used. The needle is advanced until blood flashback confirms needle position.

Subclavian vein

Infraclavicular approach: the needle is inserted below the clavicle at the junction between its medial and middle thirds. Needle is advanced medially and upwards behind the clavicle aiming towards the suprasternal notch to puncture the subclavian at its junction with IJV. The line is inserted using the Seldinger technique, and advanced into the brachiocephalic vein.

Chapter 33 **Special areas of the neck**

The neck is an anatomically crowded region, and by convention it is compartmentalized to ease understanding and communication. These conventions, which readily lend themselves to examination topics, can be intimidating; however, if they are addressed in a systematic manner they can be easily understood.

33.1 Neck fascia

Neck structures are compartmentalized by three fascial layers: **cervical; superficial,** and **deep** (Fig. 33.1).The fascia separates and supports the viscera and allows structures in the neck to move and pass over each other easily, e.g. when turning the head or swallowing (Fig. 33.2).

Superficial cervical fascia

↗ Lies between dermis and the investing layer of deep cervical fascia

↗ Contains cutaneous nerves, blood vessels, lymphatics, fat, and **platysma** anterolaterally

Deep cervical fascia

Deep cervical fascia is divided into:

↗ Investing fascia

↗ Pretracheal fascia

↗ Prevertebral fascia

Investing deep cervical fascia

↗ Most superficial layer of deep fascia

↗ Surrounds entire neck

↗ At the four 'corners' of the neck it splits into superficial and deep layers to invest the **trapezius** and **SCM**

↗ Arises from the skull superiorly: superior nuchal line of occipital bone; mastoid processes of temporal bones; zygomatic arches; inferior mandible; hyoid and spinous processes of cervical vertebrae

↗ Attaches to scapular spine, acromion and clavicle inferiorly

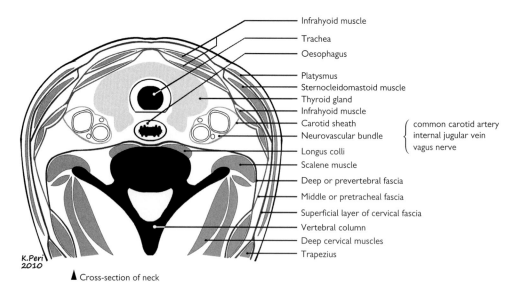

Infrahyoid muscle
Trachea
Oesophagus

Platysmus
Sternocleidomastoid muscle
Thyroid gland
Infrahyoid muscle
Carotid sheath — { common carotid artery
Neurovascular bundle — internal jugular vein
vagus nerve
Longus colli
Scalene muscle
Deep or prevertebral fascia
Middle or pretracheal fascia
Superficial layer of cervical fascia
Vertebral column
Deep cervical muscles
Trapezius

K.Peri
2010

▲ Cross-section of neck

Fig. 33.1 Cross-section of the neck showing fascial layers.

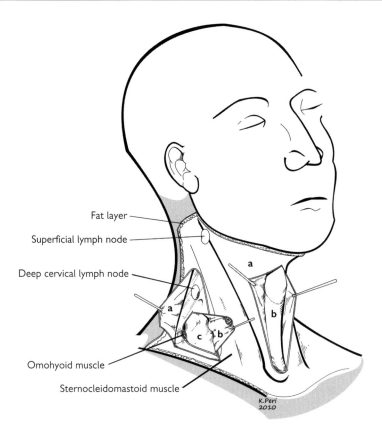

a Superficial layer of cervical fascia
b Middle or pretracheal fascia
c Deep or prevertebral fascia

Fig. 33.2 Fascias of the neck.

Pretracheal deep cervical fascia

⤢ Anterior neck only

⤢ Extends inferiorly from hyoid bone into the thorax, where it merges with the fibrous pericardium

⤢ Includes a thin muscular layer enclosing the thyroid gland, trachea, and oesophagus

⤢ Continuous laterally into the carotid sheaths

⤢ Continuous posteriorly with the buccopharyngeal fascia of the pharynx

Prevertebral deep cervical fascia

⤢ Forms a tubular sheath for the vertebral column and associated muscles, i.e. longus colli and capitus anteriorly, scalene laterally, deep cervical muscles posteriorly

⤢ Extends from base of skull to T3 vertebra (merges with anterior longitudinal ligament)

⤢ Extends laterally as axillary sheath (surrounding axillary vessels and brachial plexus)

How might the deep fascia influence the spread of infection from the neck?

↗ Fascial layers determine the direction in which a neck infection may spread. The investing layer of deep cervical fascia prevents the spread of abscesses.

↗ Infection between the investing and pretracheal deep cervical fascia can spread inferiorly to the thoracic cavity anterior to the **fibrous pericardium.**

↗ Pus from an abscess posterior to the prevertebral deep cervical fascia can extend laterally, causing swelling **posterior to SCM.**

33.2 Neck muscles

There are three key superficial neck muscles that divide the neck in to anatomical triangles: **platysma, sternocleidomastoid,** and **trapezius.** Understanding these muscles is key to understanding neck anatomy.

Platysma

↗ Thin sheet of muscle running from mandible to pectoral muscle

↗ Innervated by **facial nerve (CN VII)**

↗ Draws down corners of mouth

Sternocleidomastoid

↗ SCM is key muscle to understanding neck anatomy, as it divides neck into anterior and posterior triangles and is key landmark

↗ Runs from mastoid to **manubrium** and **clavicular head**

↗ Innervated by **accessory nerve (CN XI)**

↗ Rotates head

Trapezius

↗ Massive muscle at posterior of neck and thorax

↗ Runs from origins on occiput and spinous processes, cervical and thoracic vertebrae

↗ Inserts into scapular and clavicle

↗ Innervated by **accessory nerve (CN XI)**

↗ Elevates scapula (shrugs shoulder)

33.3 Triangles of the neck

To facilitate anatomical description, on each side, the neck is divided into two triangles, **anterior** and **posterior,** by the oblique SCM (Fig. 33.3).

For more precise localization of structures, the posterior triangle is divided into **supraclavicular** and **occipital** triangles by the inferior belly of the **omohyoid muscle.**

The anterior triangle is divided into the **submental** triangle (unpaired), **submandibular, carotid,** and **muscular** (paired) triangles by the **digastric** and **omohyoid** muscles.

Posterior triangle

Anterior	Posterior edge of SCM
Posterior	Anterior edge of trapezius
Base	Medial third of clavicle

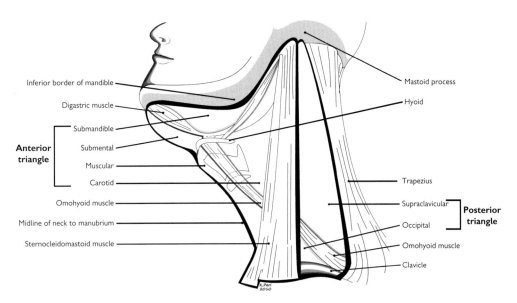

Fig. 33.3 Triangles of the neck.

Contents

↗ Accessory nerve (CN XI)

↗ Trunks of brachial plexus

↗ Lymph nodes

> Very common examination topics:
> ↗ What are the boundaries of the posterior triangle?
> ↗ What are the contents of the posterior triangle? (Fig. 33.4)
> ↗ What layers would you pass through to reach these structures? (Fig. 33.5, Fig. 33.6)

Anterior triangle

Posterior   Anterior edge of SCM

Anterior   Midline

Roof   Inferior border of mandible

Contents (Fig. 33.7, Fig 33.8)

↗ Carotid sheath

↗ Anterior jugular veins

↗ Lymph nodes

↗ Thyroid

↗ Larynx and pharynx

↗ Anterior neck strap muscles (i.e. sternothyroid and sternohyoid)

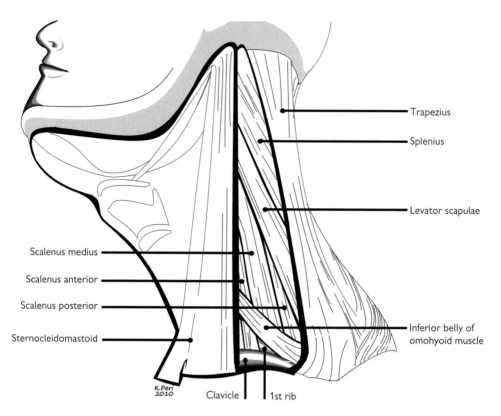

Fig. 33.4 Muscles of the posterior triangle of the neck.

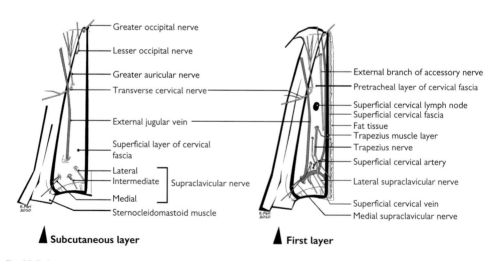

Fig. 33.5 Superficial layer of posterior triangle of the neck.

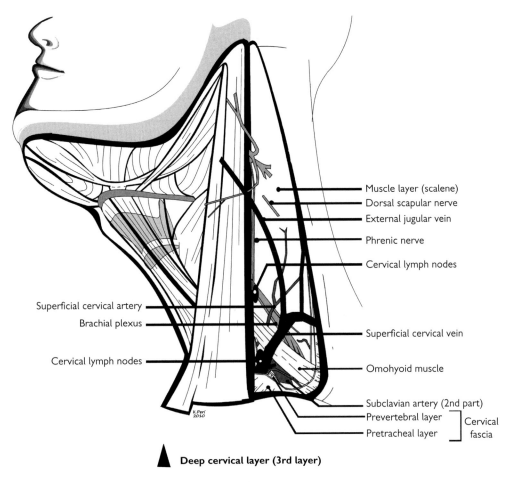

Fig. 33.6 Deep layer of the posterior triangle of the neck.

33.4 Surface anatomy of the neck

External jugular vein (EJV)

⤢ Usually visible as it crosses the neck obliquely, deep to platysma and superficial to SCM

Subclavian artery

⤢ Palpate inferoposteriorly from the posterior margin of the medial and lateral thirds of the clavicle

Submandibular lymph nodes

⤢ Palpate between the mandible and the submandibular gland

Submental lymph nodes

⤢ Under the chin

Hyoid

⤢ Anterior neck in the deep angle between the mandible and thyroid cartilage at the level of C3

⤢ Moves on swallowing

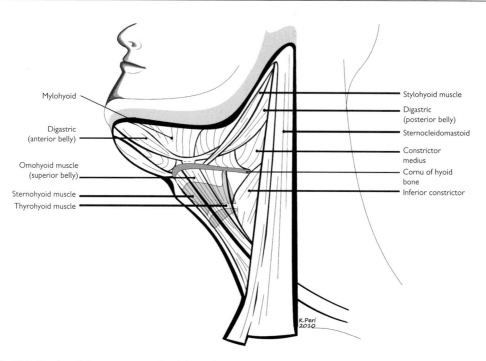

Mylohyoid

Digastric
(anterior belly)

Omohyoid muscle
(superior belly)

Sternohyoid muscle
Thyrohyoid muscle

Stylohyoid muscle

Digastric
(posterior belly)

Sternocleidomastoid

Constrictor
medius

Cornu of hyoid
bone

Inferior constrictor

K.Peri
2010

Fig. 33.7 Muscles of the anterior triangle of the neck.

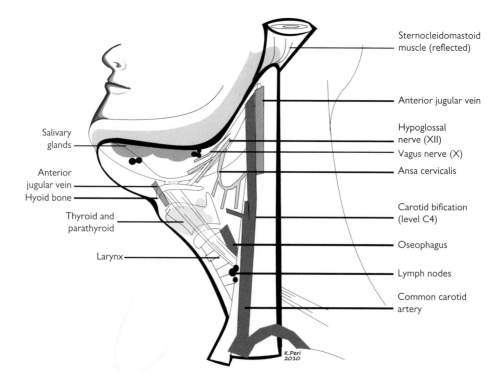

Salivary
glands

Anterior
jugular vein
Hyoid bone

Thyroid and
parathyroid

Larynx

Sternocleidomastoid
muscle (reflected)

Anterior jugular vein

Hypoglossal
nerve (XII)
Vagus nerve (X)

Ansa cervicalis

Carotid bification
(level C4)

Oseophagus

Lymph nodes

Common carotid
artery

K.Peri
2010

Fig. 33.8 Contents of the anterior triangle of the neck.

Laryngeal prominence

↗ At the meeting of the laminae of the thyroid cartilage at an acute angle in the anterior midline

↗ Recedes on swallowing

Carotid pulse

↗ Palpate the thyroid cartilage and then posterolaterally between the trachea and SCM

Cricoid cartilage

↗ Felt inferior to the laryngeal prominence (**thyroid cartilage**) at C6 level. Indicates junction of trachea and larynx and junction of pharynx and oesophagus

↗ Point at which the RLN enters the larynx—3 cm superior to thyroid gland. Immediately superior you can feel the cricothyroid ligament (site for needle/surgical cricothyroidotomy)

Cervical vertebrae

C1

↗ Tubercles can be palpated by deep pressure, postero-inferior to the tips of the mastoid processes

C6, C7

↗ Spinous processes are palpable and visible especially when the neck is flexed

One of the ways anatomy is examined is with an actor 'live model'. Make sure you can locate all these landmarks on a living subject as well as on a prosected specimen.

33.5 Anatomical zones of the neck

Zone I

↗ Root of neck from the clavicles and manubrium to the inferior border of thyroid cartilage

↗ Vulnerable structures include cervical pleurae, lung apices, thyroid, parathyroid, trachea, oesophagus, jugular veins, and cervical vertebrae

Zone II

↗ Cricoid cartilage to angles of the mandible

↗ Vulnerable structures include thyroid, larynx, carotids, jugular veins, oesophagus, and cervical vertebrae

Zone III

Angles of the mandible superiorly. Vulnerable structures include oropharynx and oral and nasal cavities

Injuries in **zones I and III** obstruct the airway and have the greatest morbidity and mortality. This is because injured structures are difficult to visualize and repair; also, vascular damage is harder to control by direct pressure in comparison with **Zone II.**

33.6 Root of the neck

The root of the neck is the junction between the thorax and neck where structures pass from the head to the thorax and vice versa.

Boundaries

Lateral   1st ribs and costal cartilages

Anterior   Manubrium

Posterior   Body of T1

Contents

Arteries   Brachiocephalic trunk (right), CCA, and subclavian (left)

Veins   Anterior jugular and IJV form brachiocephalic vein and EJV/subclavian vein

Nerves   Vagus, RLN, phrenic, sympathetic trunks, and cervical sympathetic ganglia

33.7 Carotid sheath

Carotid sheath is covered by fascial layers from the base of the skull to the root of the neck. This is continuous anteriorly with the investing and pretracheal deep cervical fascia

It communicates freely (e.g. for spread of infection and blood) with the thoracic mediastinum inferiorly and the cranial cavity superiorly.

Contents

↗ CCA, ICA

↗ IJV

↗ Vagus nerve CN X

↗ Deep cervical lymph nodes

↗ Carotid sinus nerve

↗ Sympathetic nerve fibres (carotid plexus)

33.8 Neck lymph nodes

All structures in the head and the neck drain into the deep cervical lymph nodes directly or ultimately.

Superficial cervical chain

↗ Drain the parotid and lower part of the ear

↗ Located vertically along the course of the EJV posterior to deep cervical chain

Deep cervical chain

↗ Located vertically along the IJV from the base of the skull to the root of the neck

↗ Drain into the jugular lymphatic ducts which enter the thoracic duct on the left and enter the junction of the IJV and subclavian vein on the right

↗ Submental, submandibular, preauricular, occipital, and mastoid groups

↗ Named according to their location

↗ Drain the superficial tissues of the head and neck

↗ Efferents then pass to the deep cervical chain

↗ Some pass direct to superficial cervical chain

Anterior cervical chain
- ↗ Includes the infrahyoid, prelaryngeal and pre- and paratracheal lymph nodes
- ↗ Drain into thyroid, trachea, and part of pharynx
- ↗ Empty into deep cervical chain

Retropharyngeal nodes
- ↗ Lie vertically posterior to the pharynx
- ↗ Drain back of the nose, pharynx, eustachian tube
- ↗ Empty into deep cervical chain
- ↗ Head and neck lymph eventually drains into inferior deep cervical lymph nodes, then into the supraclavicular nodes next to the transverse cervical artery
- ↗ Thoracic duct enters left brachiocephalic vein and drains lymph from the entire body

33.9 Nasopharynx

The nasopharynx may be visualized by a mirror passed through the mouth, or by an endoscope passed along the floor of the nose (posterior rhinoscopy). It may be palpated by a finger passed behind the soft palate during anaesthesia.

The soft palate cuts off the nasopharynx during deglutition and therefore prevents regurgitation of food through the nose. Lying superiorly to the soft palate and is the posterior extension of the nasal cavities. The nose opens into the nasopharynx through two **choanae.**

The roof and posterior wall form a continuous surface lying inferior to the sphenoid and occipital bones.

The '**adenoids**' or nasopharyngeal tonsils are a lymphoid tissue collection beneath the epithelium of the roof and posterior tonsillar wall. It forms **Waldeyer's ring,** which is a continuous lymphoid ring with the palatine tonsils and the lymphoid nodules on the dorsum of the tongue.

The adenoids are prominent in children but atrophy after puberty. When chronically inflamed they may almost completely fill the nasopharynx, causing mouth-breathing, and blocking the eustachian tube, causing deafness and otitis media.

The **eustachian canal** (auditory/pharyngotympanic tube) lies on the side wall of the nasopharynx parallel with the floor of the nose.

Section 2 Pathology and Physiology

Chapter 34 **Thyroid and parathyroid glands**

34.1 Thyroid physiology

The thyroid produces tetraiodothyronine (**T4** thyroxine) and triiodothyronine (**T3**) in response to **thyroid stimulating hormone (TSH)** released from the anterior pituitary gland (itself in response to **THRH** released from the hypothalamus). It also releases **calcitonin**, which regulates serum calcium levels.

> Thyroid is a relatively common subject and easily examined in a clinical examination station if you have chosen Head and Neck for the iMRCS. Thyroid pathology and physiology may well be examined in the same station.

T4 is the principal thyroid hormone, with a longer half-life than T3 but less potency.

T3 may also be produced by the conversion of T4 in peripheral tissues (80% of total body T3).

Reversed T3 (r-T3), an inactive thyroid hormone, may also be produced during conversion, which acts as a point of thyroid hormone control peripherally. Thyroid hormones act on intracellular receptors to activate genes in the cell nucleus.

Role of thyroid hormones

* Increased basal metabolic rate (BMR): increased energy and oxygen consumption, increased heat production
* Protein metabolism—protein degradation with hyperthyroidism but synthesis when euthyroid
* Carbohydrate metabolism: increased glycolysis, gluconeogenesis, and glycogenolysis
* Fat metabolism: increased lipolysis and oxidation of the plasma free fatty acids (FFAs) produced
* Increases cardiac output (CO): partly by increased BMR, also by enhancing action of other hormones
* Central nervous system development and increased cortical arousal
* Enhances action of other hormones, e.g. insulin and catecholamines

34.2 Thyroid endocrine abnormalities

> Consider and be prepared to discuss the causes of hypo/hyper/normal thyroid function in the context of an enlarged/normal sized thyroid in your clinical examination.

Causes of hyperthyroidism

* Common (85–90%):
  * Diffuse toxic goitre (Graves' disease), 50–60%
  * Toxic multinodular goitre (Plummer's disease)
* Less common:
  * Iodine induced thyrotoxicosis (iatrogenic, e.g. radiological investigations)
  * Overtreatment with thyroxine (iatrogenic)
  * Pregnancy
* Uncommon:
  * Pituitary tumour producing TSH
  * Excess HCG production (chorionic mole/choriocarcinoma)
  * Pituitary resistance to thyroid hormone
  * Metastatic thyroid carcinoma
  * Struma ovarii (thyroid tissue in dermoid cyst of ovary)

Graves' disease

- Hyperthyroidism with diffuse goitre
- M:F = 1:9, as autoimmune disease
- Caused by polyclonal immunoglobulins, which bind to and stimulate TSH receptors in the thyroid
- Graves' eye disease (proptosis, lid lag, lid retraction, exophthalmos)
- Exophthalmos is due to retro-orbital inflammation and lymphocytic infiltration, leading to oedema and increase in retrobulbar orbital
- Lid lag is due to sympathetic overstimulation and restrictive myopathy of levator palpebrae superioris
- Thyroid acropachy (clubbing)
- Pretibial myxoedema
- Normochromic, normocytic anaemia, increased ESR, and hypercalcaemia may also occur
- Associated with other autoimmune diseases

Look out for other signs of hyperthyroidism (? Graves') and hypothyroidism as part of your Head and Neck clinical examination station.

Treatment

Medical

- Antithyroid drugs, e.g. carbimazole, methimazole, propylthiouracil (inhibit thyroid peroxidase)
- Beta-blockers, e.g. propranolol (reduce effects of excess circulating thyroxine)

Radio-iodine

- Treatment of choice (pregnancy and lactation absolute contraindications)
- Single oral dose of iodine-131 directly damages replication of thyroid follicular cells
- Complications: early/late hypothyroidism, late hyperparathyroidism

Surgical

- Bilateral subtotal thyroidectomy
- Useful if patient is pregnant or wishing to become pregnant within 4 years, <30 years old, or if nodular/large goitre
- Eye signs may not regress postoperatively and may temporarily worsen
- Patient rendered euthyroid preoperatively, e.g. using carbimazole
- Oral iodine 1 mg OD for 10 days reduces gland vascularity and theoretically blood loss

Conservative

- Remove goitrogens, e.g. cabbage, from diet
- 100–300 µg thyroxine/day induces regression in up to 70% (as size of MNG is TSH dependent)
- Thyrotoxicosis, treat as Graves' disease
- Aspirate cysts (and cytology); if recurrent, instil tetracycline
- Radio-iodine (if unfit for surgery)

Remember to structure all of your answers to show that you fully understand the topic and can think through an answer logically, e.g. splitting treatment into surgical, medical, or conservative subsections.

34.3 Goitre

A goitre is any swelling of the thyroid gland; it is usually visible when 3 × normal size.

- Diffuse goitre:
  - Graves' disease
  - Simple colloid goitre
  - Thyroiditis (Hashimoto's/de Quervain's/Riedel's)
- Multinodular goitre (MNG)
- Solitary thyroid nodule

Simple colloid goitre

- Most common thyroid abnormality
- Secondary to hyperplasia to meet physiological demand for thyroxine
- Causes:
  - Iodine deficiency
  - Increased thyroxine demand (puberty, pregnancy, lactation)
  - Goitrogens, e.g. raw cabbage, lithium
  - Iatrogenic hypothyroidism
  - Defects of thyroid hormone production

Multinodular goitre (MNG)

- Progression from simple diffuse goitre to nodular enlargement
- Most common in middle-aged women
- Malignant change occurs in 5%
- May be mildly hyperthyroid (Plummer's syndrome)
- No ophthalmic symptoms

Solitary thyroid nodule

Causes

- Prominent nodule in a multinodular goitre
- Cyst (haemorrhage into necrotic nodule)
- Adenoma
- Carcinoma/lymphoma
- Thyroiditis

Features

- F:M = 4:1
- Most common in 4th and 5th decades
- 10% malignant in middle aged patients but 50% malignant in young and elderly
- FNAC most important investigation; if benign, leave alone, if malignant, surgical excision
- Technetium radio-isotope scans differentiate hot (5% malignant) from cold nodules (20% malignant)
- Cold nodules that are partly cystic/solid are considered malignant until proven otherwise

Investigations

- Clinical examination, FNAC, and technetium radio-isotope scan

Treatment

Depends on investigation results

↗ Hot nodule, patient euthyroid—FNAC (if benign, watch; if malignant, excise)

↗ Hot nodule, patient hyperthyroid—partial thyroidectomy/radio-iodine

↗ Cold nodule, true cyst—FNAC and watch

↗ Solid/partly cystic—thyroidectomy

34.4 Thyroid malignancy

Classification

↗ Five main types:

- Papillary (75%)
- Follicular (10%)
- Medullary (8%)
- Anaplastic (5%)
- Thyroid lymphoma (2%)

↗ Low incidence: 4 per 100,000 per year

↗ All types of thyroid carcinoma except follicular can be diagnosed on FNAC

↗ Differential diagnosis:

- Follicular adenoma
- Dominant nodule in a multinodular gland
- Colloid nodule
- Enlarged intrathyroid parathyroid gland

Histological demonstration of capsule invasion/peripheral vessels confirms histological diagnosis.

Prognosis

↗ Males have a poorer prognosis than females except in thyroid lymphoma

↗ Increased age, higher grade, and extrathyroidal spread in nonpapillary tumours are all poor prognostic indicators

Papillary carcinoma

↗ Occurs in young, M:F = 1:2

↗ Incidental diagnosis ≤5% post-mortems

↗ ≤50% multifocal

↗ Early spread to local lymph nodes (lymph node metastasis in 50% small tumours and 80% of large tumours)

↗ Late haematogenous spread

↗ May be related to radiation exposure (iatrogenic or nuclear power plants)

↗ Distinctive histological appearance

↗ Treatment by total thyroidectomy and resection of palpable nodes

↗ Postoperative high-dose thyroxine suppresses TSH

↗ Radio-iodine may be used to ablate any remaining thyroid tissue

↗ 90% 5 year survival rate

Follicular carcinoma

- ↗ Mean age of onset 50 years
- ↗ Rare as incidental finding
- ↗ Rarely multifocal
- ↗ Unrelated to radiation exposure, increased incidence in iodine-deficient areas
- ↗ Often metastasizes early via blood to bone marrow and lungs (lymph node metastasis unusual)
- ↗ Bland histological appearance—diagnosis depends on behaviour, i.e. capsular invasion or angiogenesis and tumour periphery
- ↗ Treatment by total thyroidectomy ± radio-iodine
- ↗ 70% 5-year survival rate (50–100% depending on metastasis)

Medullary carcinoma

- ↗ Derived from calcitonin-producing thyroid C cells, which stain apple-green with Congo red (therefore contain amyloid)
- ↗ Lymph node and bone marrow metastasis
- ↗ Up to 20% associated with multiple endocrine neoplasia type II (MEN II)
- ↗ Spontaneous (80%) usually unilateral; if genetically determined usually bilateral
- ↗ Treatment is total thyroidectomy (curative if no metastasis)
- ↗ Overall 60% 5-year survival

Anaplastic carcinoma

- ↗ Usually in elderly patients with rapidly growing tumours and pressure-related symptoms
- ↗ Associated with iodine deficiency
- ↗ Associated with pre-existing thyroid disease, e.g. multinodular goitre
- ↗ Early metastasis to local and distant sites via blood and lymphatics
- ↗ Distinctive histological appearance (sheets of highly mitotic and atypical cells)
- ↗ Treatment by debulking surgery and radiotherapy (palliative)
- ↗ 0% 5-year survival rate (10% 3-year survival rate)

Thyroid lymphoma

- ↗ Nearly always non-Hodgkin's lymphoma (NHL)
- ↗ NHL may be associated with Hashimoto's disease (and Graves')
- ↗ Two main types: aggressive (most)/indolent
- ↗ 3% of all NHL are thyroid NHL
- ↗ 5% of all thyroid carcinomas are NHL
- ↗ Indolent type is associated with mucosa associated lymphoid tissue (MALT)
- ↗ FNA may resemble anaplastic carcinoma or lymphocytic thyroiditis
- ↗ Treatment: chemotherapy gives good results (surgical excision not indicated)
- ↗ 85% 5-year survival rate

Surgical treatment of carcinoma

- ↗ Bilateral subtotal thyroidectomy with postoperative thyroxine replacement
- ↗ Total thyroidectomy avoided because of risk to recurrent laryngeal nerve (RLN) and parathyroids

↗ Indications for surgical excision:

- Obstruction (e.g. dysphagia)
- Cytological features/strong suspicion of malignancy
- Cosmesis
- Thyrotoxicosis and failed medical management

34.5 Thyroid status

Clinical features

Hyperthyroidism	Hypothyroidism
Decreased appetite	Increased appetite
Loss of weight	Weight gain
Irritability, insomnia, anxiety, emotional lability, psychosis	Lethargy, depression; slow speech, thought, and actions
Heat intolerance	Cold intolerance
Increased perspiration	Dry, peaches and cream complexion
	Hair loss (especially lateral 1/3 eyebrows)
Muscle fatigue/tremor	Proximal muscle wasting and weakness
Tachycardia, atrial fibrillation	Bradycardia
Diarrhoea	Constipation
Menorrhagia	Oligo/amenorrhoea
Fine tremor	Carpal tunnel syndrome

Thyroid function tests (TFTs)

↗ Usually TSH only, ± T3, T4 if TSH is abnormal; may include calcitonin

↗ Thyroid autoantibodies are nonspecific for thyroid autoimmune disease

Fine needle aspiration cytology (FNAC)

↗ Determines whether cystic/solid lump

↗ Provides sample for histological diagnosis

↗ Possible results:

- Benign
- Papillary carcinoma
- Follicular cells
- Thyroiditis
- Lymphoma
- Insufficient sample

Ultrasound scan

↗ Morphology of gland, i.e. solid or cystic

↗ Not sensitive/specific for thyroid malignancy (as incidence of carcinoma in cysts, solitary lumps, and multinodular glands is similar)

CT scan
- ↗ Defines relationship of thyroid to trachea, retrosternal progression and any lymphatic involvement if suspect malignancy

34.6 Thyroid gland surgery

Consent and complications of thyroidectomy

> Complications of any surgical procedure are discussed in terms of whether they are general to all operations, e.g. infection and anaesthetic, or specific problems. Complications are then further divided into immediate, early, and late. This is a recurring question in the MRCS examination.

- ↗ General:
  - Infection
  - Scar
- ↗ Specific:
  - Immediate (<24 hours):
    - ≡ Haemorrhage-expanding haematoma may lead to airway obstruction, therefore suture cutters should be next to the patient's bed postoperatively
    - ≡ Hoarseness due to damage to RLN—5% incidence (neurapraxia causes temporary hoarseness)
    - ≡ Hyperthyroidism—if severe is known as a thyroid storm
  - Early (<30 days):
    - ≡ Infection
    - ≡ Hypoparathyroidism
    - ≡ Leading to hypocalcaemia (temporary/permanent), therefore check calcium levels postoperatively
  - Late (>30 days):
    - ≡ Hyper- or hypothyroidism
    - ≡ Hypertrophic scarring/normal scarring ± surrounding numbness

34.7 Parathyroid physiology

Effects of parathyroid hormone (PTH):
- ↗ Mobilizes calcium from bone
- ↗ Enhanced calcium absorption from small intestine
- ↗ Suppresses calcium loss from kidneys
- ↗ All act to increase plasma calcium level via feedback mechanism

34.8 Parathyroid pathology

Hyperparathyroidism classification

Primary	Benign adenoma (occasionally parathyroid hyperplasia, rarely carcinoma)
Secondary	Renal failure (failure to excrete phosphate and reabsorb calcium, causing high phosphate and low calcium, and bone decalcification
Tertiary	Autonomous hypersecretion of PTH following chronic hypocalcaemia which results in hypercalcaemia

Clinical features

'Moans, stones, and groans' are features of hyperparathyroidism.

Moans   Various neuropsychiatric disorders

Stones   Increased renal calculi

Abdominal groans   Abdominal pain, constipation, pancreatitis, vague abdominal symptoms

Diagnosis

↗ Persistently high serum calcium and PTH (or PTH that is inappropriately normal in the presence of high serum calcium)

Parathyroidectomy

↗ Reverses bone decalcification, depression, anxiety, and some cardiac changes

↗ Serum calcium >3 mmol/L is an indication for surgery

↗ Preoperative treatment with 1α-hydroxycholecalciferol prevents 'hungry bone syndrome' postoperatively by minimizing catastrophic falls in serum calcium (thus reducing cardiac arrhythmias)

↗ Define parathyroid glands

↗ Remove single enlarged gland. If all four are enlarged, remove 3½

Chapter 35 **Pituitary physiology and pathology**

35.1 Pituitary physiology

The anatomy and physiology of the pituitary–hypothalamic axis are summarized in Fig. 35.1.

Adenohypophysis (anterior pituitary)

The pituitary is connected to the hypothalamus via the pituitary portal system of blood vessels, through which hypothalamic releasing and inhibiting hormones are transported.

In response to releasing hormones from the **hypothalamus,** i.e.

* **GHRH** (growth hormone releasing hormone)
* **ACRH** (adenocorticotropin releasing hormone)
* **TRH** (thyroid releasing hormone)
* **PRLRH** (prolactin releasing hormone)
* **GnRH** (gonadotropin releasing hormone)
* **POMC** (pro-oiomelanocortin)

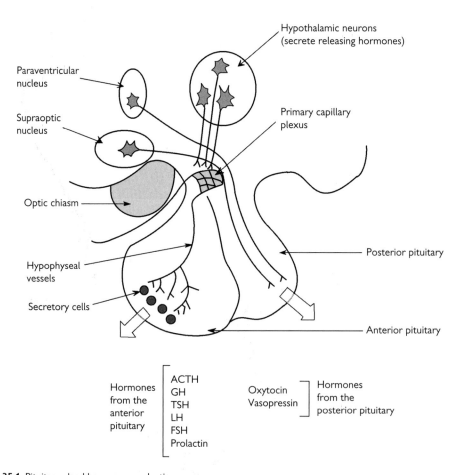

Fig. 35.1 Pituitary gland hormone production.

the **adenohypophysis** produces:

GH (growth hormone, somatotropin)	Body growth, stimulates secretion of IGF-1
ACTH (corticotropin)	Stimulates secretion and growth of zona fasciculata and reticularis of adrenal cortex
TSH (thyrotropin)	Stimulates thyroid secretion and growth of thyroid gland
PRL (prolactin)	Stimulates secretion of milk and maternal behaviour
FSH (follicle stimulating hormone)	Stimulates ovarian growth/spermatogenesis
LH (luteinizing hormone)	Stimulates ovulation and luteinization of ovarian follicles/testosterone secretion
MSH (melanocyte stimulating hormone)	Stimulates melanin synthesis in melanocytes

Neurohypophysis (posterior pituitary)

The neurohyophysis is in direct contact with the hypothalamus via neural connections.

The cell bodies of the neural cells of the neurohypophysis reside in the hypothalamus, and the hormones are transported via axons to the posterior pituitary.

The **neurohypophysis** produces:

Oxytocin	causes milk ejection and contraction of pregnant uterus
ADH (vasopressin)	promotes water retention

35.2 Pituitary tumours

Pituitary tumours form intracranial space-occupying lesions and have special features related to their endocrine function and proximity to the optic chiasm.

General features

⤢ Pituitary enlargement—may compress the optic nerve at the optic chiasm directly above, causing **bitemporal hemianopia**

⤢ Headache

Treatment

⤢ Depends on the type of tumour and its size

⤢ Large tumours can be treated with radiotherapy or surgery

⤢ Specific endocrine effects can be blocked with a variety of medication, e.g. bromocriptine for prolactinomas

⤢ These drugs often control tumour growth

Chapter 36 **Salivary gland pathology**

36.1 Unilateral parotid swelling

Intraglandular causes

- ↗ Neoplasias:
  - Benign—adenoma
  - Malignant
- ↗ Sialolithiasis/sialadenitis
- ↗ Infection—mumps, HIV
- ↗ Sarcoidosis
- ↗ Sjögren's syndrome
- ↗ Facial nerve neuroma
- ↗ Temporal artery aneurysm
- ↗ Alcoholic cirrhosis
- ↗ Diabetes mellitus
- ↗ Pancreatitis
- ↗ Acromegaly
- ↗ Malnutrition

Extraglandular causes

- ↗ Lipoma
- ↗ Sebaceous cyst
- ↗ Dental infection
- ↗ Masseter hypertrophy
- ↗ Winged mandible/transverse process atlas
- ↗ Pharyngeal tumours

Investigation

- ↗ Sialogram
- ↗ FNAC
- ↗ MRI

36.2 Salivary tumours

80% of salivary gland tumours are in the parotid gland: 80% of these are benign, with 80% of these benign parotid tumours pleomorphic adenomas.

Types

- ↗ Mucoepidermoid tumour is the most common malignancy (usually in parotid gland)
- ↗ Adenoidcystic is the most common malignancy in other salivary glands
- ↗ 10% submandibular (more likely to be malignant than tumours in other glands)
- ↗ Radiation exposure only known risk factor

Clinical features suggesting malignancy

- ↗ Rapid growth and pain
- ↗ Hyperaemic, hot skin
- ↗ Craggy

⤢ Tethered to skin and underlying muscle

⤢ Irregular

⤢ Facial nerve involved (suggests invasion)

Treatment

⤢ Complete surgical excision with facial (parotid) or hypoglossal and lingual nerve (submandibular) preservation

⤢ May need adjuvant radiotherapy

36.3 Infection and inflammation

Parotid/salivary abscess

⤢ Bacterial infection localized in (parotid) gland

⤢ May result from extremely poor dental hygiene and spread to gland via ducts

⤢ Pain, erythema, fluctuant, swelling located inside parotid gland

Parotiditis

⤢ Inflammation of parotid gland

⤢ May be due to mumps—acute, generalized viral infection causing parotid enlargement

⤢ Painful due to enlargement of the gland within its tight, fibrous capsule

Sjögren's syndrome

⤢ Autoimmune disease (90% F >50 years of age)

⤢ Affects salivary gland due to lymphocyte mediated destruction of the exocrine glands secondary to B-cell hyper-reactivity and loss of suppressor T-cell activity

⤢ Associated with recurrent/constant swelling of salivary gland(s)

⤢ Patients have two of the triad of keratoconjunctivitis (dry eyes—Schirmer's test), xerostomia (dry mouth), associated connective tissue disorders, e.g. rheumatoid arthritis (50%), scleroderma, systemic lupus erythermatosus (SLE), polyarteritis nodosa (PAN), or polymyositis

⤢ Treatment: systemic steroids, artificial tears and saliva, follow-up in case of lymphoma

36.4 Salivary calculi

Definition

Salivary calculi, stones, or **sialolithiasis** all refer to the formation of hard deposits within salivary gland or ducts.

⤢ Calculi are predominantly comprised of calcium phosphate salts and cellular debris

⤢ 90% occur in submandibular gland, then sublingual, and finally the parotid, which is rarely affected because of the serous nature of its secretion

Presentation

⤢ Typically occur in teenagers or young adults

⤢ Pain, intermittently, often corresponds to saliva production when eating, as the calculus impacts within the duct (Wharton's duct—submandibular)

⤢ May present with grossly swollen salivary gland with features of infection if gland has become infected, i.e. **sialadenitis**

⤢ May occur in someone who is dehydrated or on diuretics

Investigations

- ✗ Plain radiograph will reveal 80% of calculi
- ✗ USS can provide quick and easy confirmation of the diagnosis
- ✗ **Sialograms** can define position of blockage within duct
- ✗ CT often used if surgery is contemplated

Treatment

- ✗ The calculi may be allowed to work themselves out of the duct, possible with the assistance of massage
- ✗ Calculi might be removed via the duct in a **sialotomy**
- ✗ Open surgery is rarely required

Section 3 **Clinical**

Chapter 37 Clinical stations

37.1 Skin lumps

Accurate description of skin lesions is almost as important as final diagnosis. Examination follows the standard pattern of inspection, palpation, and if appropriate (rarely) percussion and auscultation.

History features

↗ Symptoms, duration (sudden/gradual onset)

↗ Change in colour, size, bleeding, itching?

↗ History of trauma/bite/contact?

↗ Similar lesions elsewhere?

↗ Ask how it affects their life

Examination

Inspection (6S + C)	• Site, relative to bony landmark
	• Size (mm or cm, not 'pea-sized' or other vague descriptions)
	• Shape
	• Symmetry
	• Skin changes (+ surrounding)
	• Scars
	• Colour
Palpation (3T, 3F + SECCP)	• Temperature
	• Tenderness
	• Transillumination
	• Fluctuation (small lumps)
	• Fluid thrill (large lumps)
	• Fixation—decide plane by determining attached structures, e.g. skin/muscle
	• Surface—smooth/irregular
	• Edge—well/poorly defined
	• Consistency—soft/firm/hard
	• Compressibility (e.g. AVM)/reducibility (e.g. hernia)
	• Pulsatility - differentiate expansile from transmitted pulsatility
Percussion	Dull (solid)/resonant (air-filled)
Auscultation	Bruits/bowel sounds

End by say that you would like to:

↗ Examine draining lymph nodes

↗ Assess the neurovascular status of the area/limb

↗ Look for similar lumps elsewhere

↗ Do a general examination (if necessary)

37.2 Skin ulcers

Approach similarly to skin lesion but also use **BEDD:**

Base	Granulation tissue/slough/malignant change
Edge	• Sloping (healing, usually venous/traumatic)
	• Punched out (ischaemic/neuropathic, rarely syphilitic)
	• Undermined (pressure necrosis or TB)
	• Rolled (BCC)
	• Everted (SCC)

Depth   Which structure visualized at base? e.g. fascia, muscle, bone

Discharge *Serous, sanguinous, serosanguinous, purulent*

37.3 Neck lumps

Ensure neck is exposed down to clavicles, remove jewellery, and do not forget to examine neck from in front and behind.

Examination

Inspection
- Site, e.g. triangle/midline
- As for lump (size, shape, symmetry, skin changes, scars, colour)

Manoeuvres
- Protrusion of tongue—if lump moves, likely **thyroglossal cyst** (as related to base of tongue via tract running through hyoid bone)
- Swallowing—if lump moves up and down, it is likely to be of thyroid origin i.e. **thyroglossal cyst**

Palpation
- From behind
- Describe location of lump (which triangle?)
- Solid/cystic?
- If lump is midline, regard as **thyroid**
- If no lump found, palpate for **lymph nodes** and **salivary glands**

Differential diagnosis

Position	Solid	Cystic
Midline	Thyroid swelling	Thyroglossal cyst
Anterior triangle	Lymphadenopathy	Branchial cyst
	Chemodectoma (carotid body)	Cold abscess (TB)
Posterior triangle	Lymphadenopathy	Pharyngeal pouch
		Cystic hygroma
Within SCM	SCM tumour	

Chapter 38 Common neck lump cases

It is very common in the Head & Neck clinical part of the examination to be asked to examine a lump. You may be asked to examine the scalp, face, or neck, during which you should check carefully for a swelling. It is important to use the general lump examination template, but then to consider specific diagnoses. Go through the examination methodically so that you can give a good description of the lump, then go on to answer questions.

Remember:

⤴ **Cyst**—an abnormal sac containing gas, fluid, or semisolid material, with an epithelial lining

⤴ **Sinus**—a blind-ending track, typically lined by epithelial or granulation tissue, which opens onto an epithelial surface

⤴ **Fistula**—an abnormal communication between two epithelial surfaces (or endothelial, e.g. AV fistula)

38.1 Branchial cyst

Definitions

- ↗ Develops due to a failure of fusion of the embryonic 2nd and 3rd branchial arches
- ↗ An alternative theory is that it is an acquired condition due to cystic degeneration in cervical lymphatic tissue
- ↗ Epithelial lining
- ↗ Usually presents in a young adult in the 3rd decade
- ↗ M/F 1:1

Examination

Inspect
- Anterior triangle of the neck in front of the upper or middle third of SCM
- May have branchial fistula running between the tonsillar fossa and anterior border of SCM

Palpate
- Smooth, firm ovoid swelling
- Fluctuant
- May be hard and tethered to surrounding structures if established or recurrent infection

Tests Opaque (on transillumination)

Present

'On inspection, I can see a smooth swelling with no surface changes. On palpation I can confirm that it is located in the anterior triangle of the neck. It is approximately 2 cm diameter, and is a smooth, oval mass which is fluctuant. It does not transilluminate. There is no skin tethering, satellite lesions, or local lymphadenopathy. Differential diagnoses include a branchial cyst, dermatofibroma, lipoma, abscess, carcinoma, melanoma, or satellite lesion.'

Likely questions

1. How would you confirm the diagnosis?

After I had taken a detailed history and performed a full examination I would perform a fine needle aspiration, when I would expect to draw off an opalescent fluid which, on microscopy, would reveal cholesterol crystals or pus.

2. What are the complications and treatment options?

- ↗ The main complication is recurrence/chronic discharging sinus
- ↗ The treatment options are either conservative of, if troublesome, surgical excision: Bonney's blue dye can be injected into the fistula/sinus to allow accurate excision
- ↗ Treat infections with antibiotics, before surgery

38.2 Dermoid cyst

Definition

A dermoid cyst is an epithelial-lined cyst deep to the skin, which may be congenital or acquired.

- ↗ **Congenital dermoid cysts** are due to developmental inclusion of epidermis along lines of fusion of skin dermatomes
  - They are therefore usually found at:
    - ≈ Medial and lateral eyebrows (internal and external angular dermoid cysts)
    - ≈ Midline of nose (nasal)
    - ≈ Midline of neck and trunk
  - More common in children/young adults

⋌ **Acquired dermoid cysts** are due to forced implantation of skin into subcutaneous tissues following an injury, e.g. fingers (adults)

- Lie deep to skin in subcutaneous tissues
- Differ from lipomas as not within fat layers, and from sebaceous cysts as not attached to skin

Examination

Inspect	• Site—can occur anywhere
	• Smooth spherical swelling
	• May be associated scar from previous injury (especially adults)
Palpate	• Soft ± fluctuation
	• Nontender

Present

'On inspection, a swelling approximately 0.5 cm in size is visible in the midline of the neck, 1 cm superior to the hyoid, with no overlying skin changes. On palpation, a smooth, spherical swelling is noted. It does not transilluminate. There is no skin tethering, satellite lesion, or local lymphadenopathy. Differential diagnoses include abscess, lipoma, branchial cyst, dermatofibroma, carcinoma, melanoma, and satellite lesion.'

Likely questions

1. How would you investigate further?

After I had taken a detailed history and performed a full examination I would request a CT scan, especially if I suspected that this was a congenital cyst. This is to define the extent of the cyst, as midline congenital cysts may communicate with CSF, therefore a bony defect must be excluded.

2. What are the treatment options?

Surgical excision is the preferred treatment.

38.3 Dermatofibroma

Definition

A dermatofibroma (or fibrous histiosarcoma) is a benign neoplasm of dermal fibroblasts. Modern theory describes it as a result of an abortive immunoreactive process initiated by dendritic cells.

Examination

Inspect	Can occur anywhere, but most common on legs of young or middle-aged women
	Smooth, small pink/brown hemispherical nodules
Palpate	Firm, woody consistency
	Fully mobile over deep tissues (as part of skin)

Present

'On inspection, a pink-brown swelling approximately 0.5 cm in size is visible in the posterior triangle of the neck, with no overlying skin changes. On palpation, a smooth, hemispherical swelling is noted. It does not transilluminate. There is no skin tethering, satellite lesion, or local lymphadenopathy. Differential diagnoses include abscess, lipoma, carcinoma, melanoma, and satellite lesion.'

Likely questions

1. What are the differential diagnoses?

⋌ Malignant melanoma

⋌ BCC

↗ Abscess

↗ Lipoma

↗ Satellite lesion

2. What are the management options?

Treatment can be conservative, but more commonly excision to allow histology to confirm the diagnosis with aggressive subsequent excision of the margins if actual diagnosis is malignant melanoma or BCC.

38.4 Cystic hygroma

Definition

↗ Congenital cystic lymphatic malformation located in the posterior triangle of the neck

↗ Consists of thin-walled, single or multiple cysts (connecting or separate) in tissues at the root of the neck

↗ May be a developmental abnormality originating from primitive lymph elements

↗ 50–65% present at birth (but may present as an adult)

Examination

Inspect	Posterior triangle
Palpate	• Lobulated
	• Cystic
	• Soft and fluctuant
	• Compressible
Test	Transilluminable
End by	Inspecting oropharynx, as large cyst may extend deep to the SCM into the retropharyngeal space

Present

'On inspection, a swelling approximately 2 cm is size is visible in the posterior triangle of the neck, at the root of the neck, with no overlying skin changes. On palpation, a lobulated, soft, fluctuant, compressible swelling is noted. It transilluminates. There is no skin tethering, satellite lesion, or local lymphadenopathy. It does not extend into the oropharynx. Differential diagnoses include abscess, carcinoma, melanoma, and satellite lesion.'

Likely questions

1. What are the possible complications of a cystic hygroma?

↗ Massive cystic hygromas can obstruct childbirth

↗ Respiratory obstruction

↗ Dysphagia

38.5 Lipoma

Definition

A lipoma is a benign tumour consisting of mature fat cells.

↗ They do not undergo malignant transformation (liposarcomas arise *de novo* in deep tissues)

↗ **Adiposis dolorosa (Dercum's disease)** is multiple, painful lipomas associated with peripheral neuropathy

Examination

Inspect
- Discoid/hemispherical
- Lobulation
- If scar present, may be recurrent

Palpate
- Lobulated surface
- Soft/firm
- If soft and large, may show fluctuation
- 'Slip sign' lipoma slips away under finger on gentle pressure
- Overlying skin freely mobile (in comparison to sebaceous cyst)
- If lipoma is in muscular layer, it disappears on muscular contraction

Present

'On inspection, a swelling approximately 3 cm in size is visible in the posterior triangle of the neck, with no overlying skin changes. On palpation, a smoothly lobulated, nonfluctuant swelling with a positive slip sign is noted. It does not transilluminate. There is no skin tethering, satellite lesion, or local lymphadenopathy. Differential diagnoses include abscess, carcinoma, melanoma, and satellite lesion.'

Likely questions

1. Do lipomas undergo malignant transformation?

No, liposarcomas arise *de novo* in older patients in deeper tissues of the lower limbs.

2. What is the treatment of lipomas?

- Nonsurgical: reassure patient lump is likely to be benign
- Excision e.g. due to pain, cosmesis, usually under local anaesthetic (unless communicates with a joint, then may require general anaesthetic)

3. Do you know of any lipoma variants/associated syndromes?

Angiolipomas	Prominent vascular compartment
Hibernomas	Consist of brown fat cells
Cowden's disease	Association of lipoma, palmoplantar keratoses, multiple facial papules, oral papillomatoses, and vitiligo, with thyroid and **gastrointestinal tract** involvement
Bannayan–Zonana syndrome	Rare autosomal dominant hamartomatous disorder, characterized by multiple lipomas, macrocephaly, and haemangiomas

38.6 Cervical lymphadenopathy

History

- General symptoms, e.g. night sweats, loss of appetite/weight
- Regional symptoms, e.g. tooth decay
- Previous medical history (e.g. tumour recurrence)
- Symptoms from lump duration, pain (e.g. on alcohol ingestion if lymphoma)
- Travel (to TB endemic areas)
- Contact with animals (cat scratch fever)
- Risk factors for HIV

Examination

Palpate • Consistency: firm, craggy or rubbery
• Solitary/multiple or matted together
• Fixation—skin tethering in TB nodes/malignancy

End by saying you would like to examine the rest of the head and neck, and breasts.

Present

'On inspection there is a 2-cm swelling in the left superficial cervical chain of lymph nodes, 5 cm from the mastoid process. On palpation it is a firm, craggy mass, tethered to the overlying skin. There are no satellite lesions and it does not transilluminate. Differential diagnoses include TB, malignancy, and lymphadenopathy.'

Likely questions

1. What are the common causes of cervical lympadenopathy?

↗ Lymphoma/leukaemia

↗ Infection:

• Bacterial—tonsillitis, TB, dental abscess

• Viral—CMV, EBV, HIV

• Protozoal—toxoplasmosis

↗ Sarcoidosis

↗ Tumours (primary/secondary)

> **Remember**: causes of cervical lymphadenopathy are **LIST**—Lymphoma/Leukaemia, Infection, Sarcoidosis, and Tumours

2. How would you investigate cervical lymphadenopathy?

After a detailed history and full examination, I would request the following:

↗ USS

↗ CT/MRI

↗ FNA—false −ve rate <10%, false +ve rate <3%

↗ Blood tests—FBC, ESR, TFTs, ACE (raised in sarcoidosis)

↗ Paul–Bunnell test for mononuclear cells in glandular fever (EBV)

↗ **May need open lymph node biopsy**

3. What are the risks associated with open lymph node biopsy?

Care must be taken in the posterior triangle not to damage accessory nerve (shoulder/arm pain, winged scapula, trapezius paralysis), or the facial nerve near parotid gland.

4. What are the treatment options?

Treatment depends on the results of the histological analysis of the biopsy:

Inflammatory	Treat as appropriate
SCC	Refer to ENT surgeon for full investigations including panendoscopy to find primary, sputum cytology and CXR (later may need block dissection)
Adenocarcinoma	Look for breast/abdominal primary
Lymphoma	Open lymph node biopsy (histology and marker studies)

5. What are the two possible dissections and what does each involve?

↗ **Block dissection** of the neck involves removal of the SCM, jugular vein, and accessory nerve

↗ **Radical neck dissection** involves clearance of all lymph nodes from mandible to clavicle, and from midline to trapezius.

38.7 Thyroid gland

A clinical case based around thyroid pathology is extremely likely to come up in the examination. Although the conditions themselves are not complex, candidates get confused by not listening to the direction of the examiner. Remember, you might be asked to assess the **thyroid gland** or the **thyroid status** or **both**.

History

↗ Ask about symptoms of hyper- and hypothyroidism

↗ Ask the patient how the thyroid mass is affecting their day-to-day life

↗ Obstructive symptoms from goitre

↗ Hoarse voice

Examination

Inspect
- Obvious midline lump
- Scars (collar incision)
- Raised JVP (neck vein obstruction due to mass effect)

Palpate
- Protrude tongue during palpation of the thyroid (check for thyroglossal cyst)
- Diffuse enlargement or nodular?
- Tracheal deviation (from large goitre)
- Lump features (location, size, shape, surface, tenderness, mobility, consistency)

Percuss Inferiorly down to sternum (retrosternal extension)

Tests
- Patient sips water during palpation of the thyroid (proving mass arises from thyroid)
- Pemberton's sign

Pemberton's sign

Patients with large retrosternal goitres develop signs of venous compression on raising their arms above their head (suffusion of the face, giddiness, or syncope—therefore mention, but do not elicit).

Present

'On inspection, there is a swelling originating from the thyroid gland, with no overlying skin changes. On palpation the thyroid is diffusely enlarged, with no nodules. There is no tracheal deviation. On percussion there is no retrosternal extension. It moves superiorly and inferiorly on swallowing, but not on protrusion of the tongue. On general examination, the patient has signs of hypothryroidism, as evidenced by bradycardia, hair loss, obesity, oedema.'

General thyroid examination is rarely required in the iMRCS, but state that you would like to do this as part of your thyroid examination if you examine a thyroid swelling.

Likely questions

1. What is a goitre and do you know of any classification systems?

A goitre refers to any swelling of the thyroid gland. Goitres become visible when the thyroid is 3 × normal size and weighs more than 50 g. There is a **WHO grading scheme** for goitres:

Grade 0   No palpable or visible goitre

Grade 1   Palpable goitre

Grade 2   Goitre visible with neck in normal position

Grade 3   Goitre visible from a distance

2. What are the different types of thyroid enlargement?

Goitres can either be described as diffusely enlarged or nodularly enlarged. Diffusely enlarged goitres in hyperthyroidism are likely due to Graves' disease and in euthyroidism due to thyroiditis, in which case goitre will be tender. Nodular enlargements can be described as solitary nodules or multiple nodular goitres

38.8 Thyroid status

The widespread effect of thyroid hormones, as described in Chapter 34, indicates the spectrum of signs that might be elicited in a thyroid status examination.

From top downwards:

Head

↗ Alopecia, loss of lateral third of eyebrows (hypothyroidism)

↗ Complexion (peaches and cream—hypothyroidism)

↗ Eye signs of Graves' disease:

- Lid lag
- Lid retraction
- Exophathalmos
- Proptosis
- Chemosis
- Ophthalmoplegia

Neck

↗ Goitre/scars

↗ JVP

Chest

↗ Bradycardia (hypothyroidism)

↗ Tachycardia/AF (hyperthyroidism)

Hands

↗ Thyroid acropachy

↗ Sweating (hyperthyroidism)

↗ Palmar erythema (hyperthyroidism)

↗ Onycholysis (Plummer's nails in MNG)

↗ Vitiligo (associated with autoimmune disorders, e.g. Graves')

↗ Fine tremor (hyperthyroidism)

Legs
- ⟋ Pretibial myxoedema (Graves' disease)
- ⟋ Proximal myopathy
- ⟋ Ankle-jerks (slow relaxing if hypothyroidism)

38.9 Salivary gland swelling

Examination

Inspect
- Scars/fistula opening (after parotidectomy)
- Facial palsy with CN VII damage after parotidectomy

Palpate
- Unilateral/bilateral swelling
- Fixed to skin or underlying muscle (clench teeth to tense masseter and make parotid more prominent)
- Palpate glands and duct openings (gloves)
- Describe in relation to site of gland, e.g. parotid between SCM and mandible, submandibular at angle of jaw between mylohyoid and mandible

Test   Inspect **Stensen's duct**, i.e. opening of parotid duct (opposite 2nd upper molar) and **Wharton's duct**, i.e. opening of submandibular duct on floor of mouth next to frenulum linguae, looking for pus, inflammation, or stone

End by offering to perform a full ENT examination **and** test facial nerve

Present

'On inspection there is an 3 cm swelling originating from the left parotid gland, i.e. along the angle of the mandible, with no overlying skin changes. On palpation there is a discrete, smooth, firm mass, not tethered to the overlying skin. There are no satellite lesions and it does not transilluminate. Stenson's duct appears normal. Differential diagnoses include salivary calculus, abscess/localized infection, malignancy, and dermoid cyst. Facial nerve is functional bilaterally.'

Likely questions

1. What are the different types of salivary gland tumour and where do they occur?

80% salivary gland tumours in parotid gland, 80% of these are benign, with 80% of these benign parotid tumours **pleomorphic adenomas**. **Mucoepidermoid tumour** is the most common malignancy (usually in parotid). **Adenoidcystic** is the most common malignancy in other salivary glands.

10% of salivary gland tumours are submandibular (twice as likely to be malignant as tumours in other glands). Radiation exposure is the only known risk factor.

Chapter 39 **Common skin cases**

It is very common in the Head & Neck clinical part of the examination to be asked to examine a skin lesion. You will normally be directed to the lesion, rather than expected to 'find' it. It is important to go through the examination methodically so that you can give a good description of the lesion, then go on to answer questions.

Common questions are the same for most lesions:

↗ Likely differentials and their aetiologies

↗ Prognosis

↗ Investigations that you would like to carry out

↗ Questions you would ask the patient

↗ Treatment

39.1 Malignant melanoma

Definition

A malignant melanoma is a carcinoma derived from melanocytes from the basal cell layer which invade the epidermis and dermis.

↗ Usually found on the legs of young women/trunk of middle-aged men

↗ Most common cancer of young adults 20–39 years

> **Remember: moles** are an excessive number of melanocytes producing a normal amount of melanin, whereas **freckles** are an excess of melanin produced by a normal number of melanocytes.

Examination

Inspect • Sun exposure
• Site (trunk/legs/sole of feet)
• Bleeding
Presence of satellite lesions

Palpate • **Raised/flush with skin**

End by examining lymph nodes

Present

'On inspection there is a 1-cm diameter pigmented lesion 2 cm superomedial to the lateral malleolus of the left leg. It is black, with irregular edges, and there are two satellite lesions at 1 o'clock and 4 o'clock. On palpation it extends approximately 0.5 cm beneath the surface of the epidermis, and is not tethered to any underlying structures. There is no local lymphadenopathy. Differential diagnoses include malignant melanoma, mole, freckle, lentigo, pigmented seborrhoeic keratosis, dermatofibroma, thrombosed haemangioma, and pigmented BCC.'

Likely questions

1. What are the differential diagnosis of malignant melanoma?

Benign differential include:

↗ Moles

↗ Freckles

↗ Lentigo

↗ Pigmented seborhhoeic keratosis

↗ Dermatofibroma

↗ Thrombosed haemangioma

Malignant differential diagnosis includes:

↗ Pigmented BCC

2. What are the features of a skin lesion that are particularly worrying?

The so-called 'red-flag' symptoms are:

↗ Ulceration

↗ Bleeding/itching

↗ Marked colour variation in lesion

↗ Halo of brown pigment/satellite nodules around the lesion

↗ Rapid increase in size/colour/thickness

3. What types of malignant melanoma do you know about?

There are four common types of melanoma:

↗ Superficial spreading melanoma (70%):
- F: legs M: backs
- Red/white/blue
- Thin but palpable
- Irregular edge

↗ Nodular melanoma (15–30%):
- Trunk
- Raised, polypoid shape
- Smooth with irregular edge
- Often ulcerated

↗ Lentigo maligna melanoma:
- Originates from lentigo maligna
- Flat, brown/black with irregular edge (thicker, darker part is malignancy)
- Affects face/dorsum hands/forearm

↗ Acral lentiginous melanoma:
- Least common
- Occurs on hairless skin (palmar hands and feet, subungal area)
- Irregular brown/black lesion

4. What are the factors that predispose to malignant melanoma?

Congenital risk factors include:

↗ Xeroderma pigmentosum

↗ Dysplastic naevus syndrome

↗ Large congenital naevi

↗ Family history (when more than one first-degree relative is affected the risk rises 50%)

↗ Fair complexion (if followed by UV exposure)

Acquired risk factors include:

↗ UV light sunlight or tanning booth

↗ Pre-existing skin lesions, e.g. lentigo maligna

↗ >20 benign pigmented naevi

↗ Previous melanoma

5. What staging systems do you know of?

The most commonly used staging systems are Clark's, Breslow's, and four-stage clinical staging systems.

Clark's system, based on invasive extent:

Level I	epidermis only	98% 5-year survival
Level II	invading papillary dermis	96% 5-year survival
Level III	fills papillary dermis	94% 5-year survival
Level IV	invading reticular dermis	78% 5-year survival
Level V	subcutaneous tissue invasion	44% 5-year survival

Breslow system is based on thickness of lesion:

<0.76 mm	93% 10-year survival
<3 mm	50% 10-year survival
<4 mm	30% 10-year survival
Lymph node involvement	<40% 8-year survival

Four-stage clinical staging system: (best prognostic indicator):

IA <0.75 mm or Clark II

IB 0.75–1.5 mm or Clark III

IIA 1.5–4.0 mm or Clark IV

IIB >4 mm or Clark V

III Lymph node metastases in one regional drainage area or >5 'in-transit' lymph vessel metastases (ones not yet reached nodes)

IV Advanced regional nodal metastases. Also metastases to other sites such as lung, liver or brain

6. What are the treatment options?

The mainstay of treatment is surgical excision. Individual lesions can be excised with the margins described by Veronesi:

<0.76 mm 1-cm margin of grossly normal tissue (to deep fascia)

0.76–1 mm 2-cm margin

>1 mm 3-cm margin

Regional lymphatic involvement is treated with block dissection.

7. What are the factors are associated with a poor prognosis?

↗ Increased Clark's level, Breslow thickness, or four-stage clinical staging system

↗ Increasing age

↗ Male

↗ Trunk, hand, scalp, or foot

↗ Ulceration

↗ Depigmentation and amelanotic melanomas

↗ High histological grade

> Malignant melanoma is the type of lump most commonly asked about in the iMRCS Head and Neck clinical station, often as a differential. Therefore be prepared to discuss malignant melanoma in detail, although you will not be expected to know the rarer lumps in as much detail (e.g. pyogenic granuloma/neurofibroma), particularly for differential diagnoses.

39.2 Sebaceous cyst

Examination

Inspect
- Smooth hemispherical swelling
- Usually solitary
- Commonly face, trunk, neck, scalp
- Half have punctum at apex

Palpation
- Smooth surface
- Firm–soft consistency
- Punctum may exhibit plastic deformation on palpation
- Attached to skin

Present

'On inspection there is a 3-cm diameter lesion on the occiput of the scalp. There is a visible punctum. On palpation it is hemispherical, with a smooth surface and firm consistency. There are no satellite lesions or local lymphadenopathy.'

Likely questions

1. What are the main complications and treatments of sebaceous cyst?

The main complications are:

↗ Infection, common, may be associated discharge

↗ Ulceration

↗ Calcification (trichilemmal cysts) hard on palpation

↗ Sebaceous horn formation (hardening of a slow discharge of sebum from a wide punctum)

↗ Malignant change (rarely)

Although the majority of sebaceous cysts can be managed conservatively if they are small and asymptomatic, they can be surgically excised to prevent recurrence.

2. What are the histological subtypes of sebaceous cyst?

↗ **Epidermal cyst**—derived from infundibular portions of hair follicles

↗ **Trichilemmal cyst**—derived from hair follicle epithelium, therefore common on scalp, often multiple, autosomal dominant inheritance

3. What is a Cock's peculiar tumour?

It is a proliferating **trichilemmal** cyst, which is usually solitary:

↗ 90% on scalp

↗ Resemble SCC clinically and histologically

↗ Rarely, malignant transformation may occur

4. What is Gardner's syndrome?

Part of the spectrum of familial polyposis coli (FAP) syndromes, including FAP, occurs ± multiple epidermal cysts, multiple osteomas of skull, and desmoid tumours

39.3 Squamous cell carcinoma (SCC)

Definition

↗ Derived from basal epidermal cells (these usually migrate superficially to form keratizing squamous layer)

↗ Full-thickness epidermal atypia (cf. basal atypia only in solar keratosis), with tumour cells infiltrating deep dermis and subcutaneous fat

↗ Well, moderately, or poorly differentiated

History

↗ Cosmetic symptoms

↗ Predisposing factors:

- Xeroderma pigmentosum (congenital)
- Environmental agents: UV light, radiation, industrial carcinogens
- Infections e.g. HPV 5, 8
- Immunosupression
- Chronic cutaneous ulceration e.g. chronic burns, chronic venous ulcers (Marjolin's ulcer)

Examination

Inspect
- Occur anywhere on face (usually the most sun-exposed)
- Red-brown (vascular) appearance
- Raised and everted edge
- May be of considerable size
- ± local erosion/central ulceration if advanced

Palpate
- Regional cervical lymphadenopathy (due to metastases/secondary infection)
- 5% metastases at presentation

Present

'On inspection there is a red-brown lesion of 1 cm diameter on the vertex of the scalp. There is central ulceration and irregular, everted edges. There are no satellite lesions or regional lymphadenopathy. Differential diagnoses include keratoacanthoma, infected sebaceous cyst, solar keratosis, pyogenic granuloma, BCC, and malignant melanoma.'

> Common questions for head and neck cancers include describing how you would differentiate between SCC, BCC, and malignant melanoma.
>
> It is also important to be able to give their excision margins and treatment.

Likely questions

1. What is the differential diagnosis of SCC?

↗ Benign:
- Keratoacanthoma
- Infected sebaceous cyst
- Solar keratosis
- Pyogenic granuloma

↗ Malignant:
- BCC
- Malignant melanoma

2. How are SCC treated?

↗ Primary lesion:
- Excision (1 cm margin)
- Mohs' staged chemosurgery with histological assessment of margins and electrodissection (for eyelids, ears, nasolabial folds, nose)
- Radiotherapy if unresectable

↗ Nodal metastasis:
- Surgical block dissection if nodes palpable/Marjolin's ulcers
- Radiotherapy

39.4 Basal cell carcinoma (BCC)

History

Predisposing factors:

↗ Congenital (rare):
- Xeroderma pigmentosa (Kaposi's disease) with defective DNA repair
- Gorlin's syndrome (see below)

⤢ Acquired (common):

- UV light (especially UVB)
- Carcinogens, e.g. smoking and radiotherapy
- Malignant transformation in lesions, e.g. naevus sebaceous

Examination

Inspect   Occur on hair-bearing sun-exposed skin of elderly people, often around the eye
Single/multiple
Raised, nodular, or cystic
Not raised, pigmented, sclerosing, cicatriacial, or superficial

Palpate   Fixation deep to skin is a sign of deep
Local invasion

End by examining for regional lymphadenopathy (but state metastasis by malignant transformation is very rare, usually only locally aggressive)

Present

'On inspection there is a 0.5-cm brown-red nodular lesion 2 cm lateral to the left nostril. It feels superficial on palpation, and there are no satellite lesions or regional lymphadenopathy.'

Likely questions

1. Tell me more about the different types of raised and unraised BCC

Raised BCC can be either nodular or cystic:

⤢ Nodular—most common, well defined, rolled, pearly edge with central ulceration

⤢ Cystic—large cystic nodule

Unraised BCC can be divided into:

⤢ Pigmented—contains melanin

⤢ Sclerosing (morphoeic)—flat/depressed, ill-defined edge, late ulceration

⤢ Cicatriacial—multiple, superficial erythematous lesions interspersed with pale, atrophic areas

⤢ Superficial—erythematous, scaly patches (differential is Bowen's disease)

2. What is the histology of BCC?

⤢ Many histological patterns

⤢ Commonly, islands and nests of basaloid cells in the dermis with high mitotic rates and peripheral pallisading and epidermal ulceration

39.5 Pyogenic granuloma

Definition

A pyogenic granuloma is a rapidly growing capillary haemangioma usually less than 1 cm diameter (neither pyogenic nor granuloma). They are commonly found on hands and face in children/young adults, and gums and lips of pregnant women.

Examination

Inspect   • Bright red/blood-encrusted hemispherical nodule
- Skin-coloured if longstanding (epithelialization)
- Sessile/pedunculated
- Associated serous/purulent discharge

Palpate • Soft
  • Slightly compressible (due to vascular origin)
  • May bleed easily

End by asking patient:

↗ Previous injury to this area?

↗ How long lump took to appear (rapid growth in a few days)

↗ How lump affects life?

Present

'On inspection there is a 0.5-cm bright red hemispherical nodule on the left cheek, 3 cm lateral to the nose, immediately inferior to the left eye. On palpation the nodule is soft and slightly compressible. There are no satellite lesions or regional lymphadenopathy.'

Likely questions

1. What are the treatment options for pyogenic granuloma?

↗ Nonsurgical—regression uncommon except unless arise during pregnancy. Can try silver nitrate sticks

↗ Surgical—excision/curettage with diathermy of base (preferred)

39.6 Seborrhoeic keratosis

Definition

Seborrhoeic keratosis is a benign overgrowth of the epidermal basal cell layer. It is also known as **senile keratosis** due to typical age of presentation.

History

Similar lesions elsewhere? (sudden onset of multiple lesions associated with **visceral malignancy,** i.e. Leser–Trelat sign)

Examination

Inspect • Found anywhere but most commonly face and trunk
  • Single/multiple
  • Round/oval
  • 'Stuck-on' appearance
  • Brown to black colour
  • Surface appears velvety/warty
  • Can be picked off skin leaving surface capillaries that bleed slightly (do not do this!)

Present

'On inspection there is a 1-cm brown, warty looking lesion on the right cheek, 2 cm lateral to the nose. On palpation the nodule is soft and velvety. There are no satellite lesions or regional lymphadenopathy.'

Likely questions

1. What is the main differential diagnosis?

Acanthosis nigricans.

2. What are the treatment options?

Nonsurgical/ superficial shaving/cautery.

3. What are the histological types of seborrhoeic keratosis?

⤢ Hyperkeratosis (thickened keratin layer)

⤢ Hyperplasia (prickle cell layer)

⤢ Hyperplasia of variably pigmented basaloid cells

39.7 Keratoacanthoma

Definition

An overgrowth of hair follicle cells producing a central plug of keratin. It grows rapidly, forming within 6 weeks and regressing after 6 weeks, leaving a depressed scar. Clinically and cytologically they appear similar to well-differentiated SCCs.

Examination

Inspect • Located on sun-exposed areas
• Dome-shaped with central crater (containing keratin)
• Normal skin colour (except central core which is brown/black due to keratin)

Palpate • Firm with hard central core
• Fully mobile over deep tissues (as occur in skin)

Present

'On inspection there is a dome-shaped lesion which is skin coloured with a central brown core. On palpation it is firm with a hard central core and no tethering to underlying tissues.'

Likely questions

1. What are the treatment options?

⤢ Nonsurgical—leave alone if asymptomatic (especially in young)

⤢ Surgical—excision (complete), with high index of suspicion for SCC in elderly patients

39.8 Papilloma

Definition

An overgrowth of all layers of the skin with a central vascular core, increasingly common with age. Also called **skin tag/fibroepithelial polyp**.

Examination

Inspect Occur anywhere, commonly face, neck, trunk, anus

Pedunculated (or sessile) swelling

Flesh coloured

Palpate Soft

End by asking patient about:

⤢ Pregnancy

⤢ Diabetes

⤢ Intestinal polyposis

⤢ Similar lumps elsewhere?

Present

'On inspection there is a pedunculated, skin coloured lesion midway along the right mandibular border. On palpation it is soft with a narrow stalk and no tethering beneath the epidermis.'

Likely questions

1. What are the treatment options?

Excise with scissors, control bleeding from central core with suture/diathermy.

PART 4
NEUROSCIENCE

Section 1 Anatomy

Chapter 40 **Basic neuroembryology**

40.1 Spinal cord

Neurulation

The nervous system is formed from the **neural plate**, an **ectodermal** thickening in the floor of the amniotic sac.

At the 3rd week of gestation the neural plate forms paired **neural folds**, which migrate and then unite to form the **neural tube**. Union of the neural tube begins in the middle of the neural fold and proceeds in both a rostral and caudal direction. The open ends of the closing neural tube, the **neuropores**, close off before the end of the 4th week.

Cells at the tip of the migrating neural folds are not incorporated into the neural tube but form the **neural crest**. They go on to form spinal and autonomic ganglion cells and Schwann cells.

Spinal nerves

The dorsal part of the neural tube, the **alar plate**, forms predominantly sensory neurons.

The ventral part of the neural tube, the **basal plate**, forms predominantly motor neurons and gives rise to the ventral nerve roots.

The dorsal and ventral roots combine to form spinal nerves.

* Spinal dysraphisms—Failure of closure of the posterior neural arch
* Myelomeningocele—Spinal cord and roots protrude through a bony defect lined with meninges and/or skin
* Meningocele—Cystic CSF-filled cavity in communication with the spinal canal through a bony defect (most commonly lumbosacral)
* Spina bifida occulta—Bony defect; affects 5–10% of the population. Cutaneous stigmata, e.g. hairy patch, may indicate an underlying defect

40.2 Brain

Cerebrum

The rostral end of the neural tube extends to form three brain ventricles (Fig. 39.1):

* Prosencephalon (forebrain)
* Mesencephalon (midbrain)
* Rhombencephalon (hindbrain)

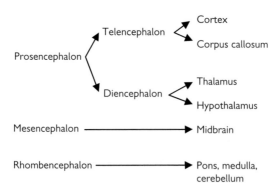

Fig. 39.1 Formation of the brain.

Cerebral hemispheres

The cerebral cortex is formed from the telencephalon.

Frontal, parietal, temporal, and occipital lobes can be identified at 14 weeks gestation.

Cells divide around the lateral ventricles and migrate outwards to form the cerebral hemispheres.

Chapter 41 Skull and meninges

41.1 Development

> Candidates are commonly handed a skull and either asked to point out features or invited to identify specific structures. The best way to prepare for the MRCS examination is with this book, an anatomical atlas, and a real skull.

The skull is formed from the membranous primordial cranium which originates from the mesoderm. This also forms the meninges, muscle, blood vessels, and skin and subcutaneous tissue of the scalp.

Bones of the base of the skull are formed from cartilage, initially divided into three segments (precordal, cordal, and prevertebral).

41.2 Sutures

The points of fusion of the bones of the skull vault are marked by the sutures, and this process continues into early childhood.

Coronal	Divides the frontal bone from the parietal bones
Sagittal	Divides the two parietal bones in the midline
Lambdoid	Marks off the occipital bone from the parietal and temporal bones
Squamosal	Separates the squamous temporal bone from the parietal bone and the sphenoid bone
Metopic	Divides the frontal bone

> **Craniosynostosis**—the premature fusion of cranial sutures leading to skull vault deformity and cranial maldevelopment in early life.

41.3 Fontanelles

Fontanelles are the 'soft spots' between unfused cranial bones which allow skull deformation during birth. Brain under the fontanelle is protected by a thick membrane. Fontanelles normally close by the age of 2 years.

Anterior fontanelle

⤢ Diamond shaped, at the junction of the sagittal and coronal sutures

⤢ Known as the **bregma** after fusion

> Puncture of the anterior fontanelle is a technique for gaining a CSF sample in an infant or accessing the sagittal sinus.

Posterior fontanelle

⤢ Triangular, at the junction of the lambdoid and sagittal sutures

⤢ Normally closes at the age of 2–3 months

> **Paranasal sinuses** form at around 8 years of age while **mastoid air cells** are seen at around 2 years.

41.4 Meninges

Meninges are comprised of three layers: the **dura mater**, **arachnoid**, and **pia mater**.

Dura mater

⤢ Formed of an outer **endosteal** layer and an inner **meningeal** layer

⤢ Attached to the skull at the cranial sutures, and so an extradural haematoma takes on a lenticular shape limited by these suture attachments

⤢ Separation of the endosteal and meningeal layers occurs to form the dural venous sinuses

⤢ Two reflections of the dura give rise to key meningeal divisions within the cranial vault:

Falx cerebri:
- Divides the two cerebral hemispheres
- Attaches anteriorly to the **crista galli** and posteriorly to the tentorium cerebelli

Tentorium cerebelli: Attaches anteriorly to the anterior and posterior clinoid processes

⤢ Between these two attachments bilaterally is the **diaphragma sellae** which lies over the sella turcica and is pierced by the pituitary stalk

⤢ Reflections of the dura give rise to the **venous sinuses**; in the middle cranial fossa the cavernous and petrosal sinuses, and in the posterior fossa the transverse sinus

Chronic subdural haematoma

Bridging veins traversing the subdural space, often fragile in old age, may be damaged during minor head trauma, giving rise to a subdural haemorrhage.

Arachnoid mater

A thin, loose layer of meninges.

The space between the dura and arachnoid mater is the **subdural space**

The **subarachnoid space** (between the arachnoid and pia mater):

⤢ Contains CSF and the major blood vessels

⤢ Extends down the spinal canal terminating at the sacrum

Small projections of arachnoid through the meningeal layer of dura at the superior sagittal sinus (the **arachnoid granulations**) are the site of CSF reabsorption.

Pia mater

A thin layer of meninges closely related to the cortical surface and conforming to the contours of the sulci and gyri (this does not occur in the cerebellum).

41.5 Base of skull

What are the signs of basal skull fractures?

- **CSF rhinorrhoea** (leakage of CSF from the nose)—a sign of an anterior cranial fossa fracture with a coexisting dural tear
- **Periorbital haematoma** (panda eyes)—also a sign of an anterior cranial fossa fracture
- **Subconjunctival haemorrhage**—caused by fracture of orbital wall
- **CSF otorrhoea**—sign of middle cranial fossa fracture
- **Battle's sign**—bruising over mastoid process appearing approximately 4 hours after a fracture in the posterior cranial fossa

Revision of this material should ideally be conducted with an anatomy atlas and skull. This section will tell you what you need to know and in what depth; you still must be able to identify these structures on a skull.

Anterior cranial fossa

This is a topic which seems to be in almost every examination in some form. The 'classic' station is where a candidate is given a skull with the cranial vault removed and invited to identify the fossae, the foramina, and the structures they transmit.

The floor of the anterior cranial fossa is formed from the orbital plate of the **frontal bone** (forming most of the anterior portion), the **ethmoid bone** (forming part of the central portion), and the **sphenoid bone** (forming the posterior portion).

The boundaries are the **frontal bone** forming the anterior and lateral walls and the **anterior clinoid process** and **tuberculum sellae** and the curved surface of the lesser wing of the **sphenoid bone** posteriorly.

Crista galli

(Latin: crest of the cock), a raised portion of the **ethmoid bone** between the cerebral hemispheres, is the area of attachment of the **falx cerebri.**

Middle cranial fossa

The floor of the middle cranial fossa is complex and contains the majority of the skull foramina through which **vessels** and **nerves** pass from the intracranial compartment.

It is formed by the **body** and **greater wing** of the **sphenoid bone** (forms the anterior portion) and the squamous part of the **temporal bone** laterally.

The petrous part of the temporal bone forms the posterior boundary.

Sella turcica

Located in the midline bound by the anterior clinoid processes and tuberculum sellae anteriorly and the dorsum sellae with posterior clinoid processes posteriorly. Contains the **pituitary gland.**

Posterior cranial fossa

Predominantly **occipital bone.** Anterior margin is the petrous part of the **temporal bone** laterally and the **clivus** (extending from the **dorsum sellae** to the anterior **foramen magnum**).

41.6 Cranial foramina

Foramina from anterior to posterior:

Cribriform plate

Found either side of the midline in the floor of the anterior part of the anterior cranial fossa. This is a very thin area of the **ethmoid bone** with multiple perforations.

Transmits: • Olfactory tracts CN I
 • Emissary veins
 • Anterior ethmoidal nerves and veins

Optic canal

Either side of the midline underneath the tuberculum sellae.

Transmits: • Optic nerves CN II
 • Ophthalmic artery

Superior orbital fissure

Lies underneath lesser wing of sphenoid.

Transmits: • Oculomotor nerve (CN III)
 • Trochlear nerve (CN IV)

> • Ophthalmic division of the abducens nerve (CN VI)
> • Superior ophthalmic vein

Foramen rotundum

Medially placed within middle cranial fossa.

Transmits: Maxillary branch of the trigeminal nerve (CN V2)

Foramen ovale

Posterolateral to the foramen rotundum.

Transmits: Mandibular branch of trigeminal nerve (CN V3)

Foramen spinosum

Posterolateral to the foramen ovale

Transmits: Middle meningeal artery

Middle meningeal artery (MMA)

↗ Enters the middle cranial fossa through the foramen spinosum

↗ Forms a groove in the inner aspect of the temporal bone as it travels up, supplying the meninges

↗ Common cause of an extradural haematoma due to a temporal bone fracture

---

Foramen lacerum

Intracranial opening of the carotid canal.

Transmits: Internal carotid artery

Internal acoustic meatus

Located in the medial aspect of both petrous temporal bones.

Transmits: • Facial nerve (CN VII)
         • Vestibulocochlear nerve (CN VIII)
         • Labyrinthine arteries

Jugular foramen

Located in the medial aspect of the posterior fossa just beneath the petrous temporal bone.

Transmits: • Glossopharyngeal nerve (CN IX)
         • Vagus nerve (CN X)
         • Accessory nerve (CN XI)
         • Sigmoid sinus
         • Inferior petrosal sinus

Hypoglossal canal

Located on the anterolateral rim of the foramen magnum

Transmits: Hypoglossal nerve (CN XII)

Chapter 42 **Cerebral topography**

42.1 Cerebral cortex

The cerebral cortex is divided into four lobes separated by two major sulci and two imaginary lines.

Lateral sulcus (or sylvian fissure)   separates the temporal lobes from the frontal lobe

Central sulcus (rolandic fissure)   separates the frontal lobe from the parietal lobe

An imaginary line from the **parieto-occipital sulcus** to a **preoccipital notch** at the lower border of the hemisphere separates the occipital lobe from the parietal lobe.

A further imaginary line drawn horizontally from the **posterior end of the sylvian fissure** to intersect with the previously described line separates the parietal lobe from the posterior temporal lobe.

> Connecting the two cerebral hemispheres is a massive band of white matter (**corpus callosum**) consisting of a genu (anterior end), a trunk, splenium (posterior part), and a rostrum connecting the genu to the anterior commissure.

Frontal lobe

Mainly concerned with intellectual activity, emotions, behaviour, and control of autonomic activity.

Primary motor cortex occupies most of the **precentral gyrus**; concerned with voluntary movement and receives afferent input from the **thalamus** and **cerebellum.**

In front of the motor cortex is the **premotor cortex** (or motor association area).

The areas representing the hand, lips, eyes, and foot are exaggerated out of proportion to the rest of the body.

Broca's speech area is situated around the posterior part of the inferior frontal gyrus of the **dominant hemisphere** and is concerned with the motor aspects of speech.

Parietal lobe

Bounded by the central sulcus anteriorly and posteriorly by the imaginary line drawn from the parieto-occipital sulcus to the posterior end of the lateral sulcus (or sylvian fissure).

Important cortical areas in parietal lobe include:

Somatic sensory cortex	Located on the postcentral gyrus. Receives afferent fibres from the thalamus. Controls all form of somatic sensation
Parietal association cortex	Controls integration of sensory stimuli with other forms of sensory information

Temporal lobe

Demarcated by the lateral (sylvian) sulcus separating it from the parietal lobe

Important cortical areas in the temporal lobe include:

Auditory cortex	Lying within the superior temporal gyros. Afferent fibres are received from the medial geniculate body
Temporal association area	This area of brain surrounding the primary auditory cortex and is concerned with integration of auditory stimuli with other sensory modalities

> Damage to the temporal association area leads to **temporal agnosia**—an inability to understand meaningful sounds such as a door bell or ringing phone.

Occipital lobe

Lies behind the partial and temporal lobes demarcated by the imaginary line between the parieto-occipital sulcus and the posterior tip of the sylvan fissure.

Visual cortex	Area surrounding the calcarine sulcus that receives its afferent fibres from the lateral geniculate body of the ipsilateral, receiving visual input from the contralateral visual field
Occipital association area	Lies anterior to the primary visual cortex and is concerned with recognition and integration of visual stimuli

42.2 Ventricular system

Cerebrospinal fluid

↗ Produced by choroid plexus located within the lateral, IIIrd, IVth ventricles

↗ A small amount of CSF is also produced in the spinal cord

↗ Total circulating CSF in adults: 150 ml

↗ CSF is produced at a rate of 450–750 ml daily

↗ Absorption takes place in the arachnoid villi which protrude into the dural venous sinuses

↗ Normal CSF pressures 8–10 cmH$_2$O

Lateral ventricles

The largest of the ventricles, lie deep within the cerebral hemispheres.

↗ Boundaries are:

- Thalamus
- Caudate nucleus
- Fornix inferiorly
- Septum pallucidum
- Corpus callosum

↗ Consist of four parts:

- **frontal** (or anterior) horns
- **body**
- **occipital** (or posterior) horns
- **temporal** (or inferior) horns

Inferior to the frontal horns is a communication between the lateral ventricles with the **IIIrd ventricle**, the **interventricular foramen** (or foramen of Monro)

The **choroid plexus** extends from the temporal (inferior) horns and extend through the body descending through the foramen of Monro to the roof of the IIIrd ventricle

IIIrd ventricle

A thin, slit-like ventricle in the midline bounded on either side by the thalamus in its upper part with the hypothalamus forming the lower part and floor.

The IIIrd ventricle communicates with the IVth ventricle through the **cerebral aqueduct** (of Sylvius).

IVth ventricle

Diamond shaped ventricle with the **pons** and **medulla** forming its anterior wall and the cerebellar hemispheres and the superior and inferior **medullary vela** forming its roof.

CSF flows out of the IVth ventricle through the **foramen of Magendie** centrally and the laterally placed **foramina of Luschka.**

In addition to the ventricles CSF flows throughout the subarachnoid space around the brain and spinal cord. The more prominent of these are referred to as **cisterns**.

42.3 Basal ganglia

Consist of the **caudate nucleus, putamen, globus pallidus,** and **claustrum**.

Putamen and globus pallidus are collectively known as the **lentiform nucleus**. The lentiform nucleus is separated from the thalamus and caudate nucleus by the internal capsule. The caudate nucleus and putamen receive afferent input from the cerebral cortex and thalamus and send efferents on to the globus pallidus. The globus pallidus in turn sends efferents to the thalamus, the red nuclei, the substantia nigra and reticular formation.

There are also communications between the basal ganglia and the visual pathways via the superior colliculi.

> The basal ganglia are located deep within the cerebral hemispheres and are involved in coordination of movement. This includes complex interconnections between several elements, the failure of which leads to a number of surgically relevant movement disorders.

Chapter 43 Intracranial vasculature

Candidates in the OSCE are commonly shown a cerebral angiogram or a prosected head and asked either to point out features or to identify specific structures.

43.1 Internal carotid artery (ICA)

Course in the neck

↗ Commences at bifurcation of common carotid artery (CCA) where its origin is dilated, forming the **carotid sinus**

↗ Initially lies lateral to the external carotid artery (ECA) then passes medially and posterior to it

↗ Ascends laterally to the pharynx with the internal jugular vein (IJV), vagus nerve, and cervical sympathetic chain

↗ Initially covered superficially by sternocleidomastoid muscle, CN XII (hypoglossal nerve), and common facial vein, then passes under posterior belly of the digastric muscle and parotid gland to the base of skull

↗ Does not give off any branches in the neck

> The carotid sinus is richly innervated by the glossopharyngeal nerve (CN IX). It acts as a chemoreceptor and pressure receptor. A rise in blood pressure causes a vagally mediated decrease in heart rate and peripheral vasodilatation, whilst a reflex increase in respiratory rate is triggered by a rise in CO_2 or fall in O_2 in the blood.

Course in the skull

At the base of the skull, ICA enters the carotid canal in the petrous temporal bone and separates from the IJV.

On entering the skull, the ICA starts a tortuous course, making six bends in all:

↗ upwards into the cavernous sinus

↗ forwards in this

↗ upwards through the roof to lie medial to the anterior clinoid process

↗ turning back on itself above the sinus

↗ then passing upwards again, lateral to the optic chiasm

↗ ending by dividing into the anterior and middle cerebral arteries

These six bends are believed to relieve pressure from the systolic blood pressure on the delicate cerebral tissue.

Branches

↗ Ophthalmic artery:

  • Originates from the ICA immediately after it emerges from the cavernous sinus, and enters the orbital foramen below and lateral to the optic nerve

  • It supplies the orbital contents and skin above the eye via the **supratrochlear** and **supraorbital** branches

  • The retina is solely supplied by its branch, the **central retinal artery**

↗ Anterior cerebral artery

↗ Middle cerebral artery

> The middle cerebral artery's cerebral branches to the internal capsule are often affected by stroke, causing contralateral sensation loss and/or motor deficit.

43.2 Vertebral artery

Course

- ↗ Crosses apex of the lung, then enters, and is transmitted by, the **transverse foramina** of vertebrae C1–C6
- ↗ Turns posteriorly and medially over the posterior **arch of the atlas** to enter the cranial cavity via the **foramen magnum**, piercing the dura mater
- ↗ Runs on the anterolateral aspect of the medulla to meet the contralateral subclavian artery and form the **basilar artery** in the circle of Willis

Important branches

- ↗ Anterior and posterior spinal arteries
- ↗ Posterior inferior cerebellar artery
- ↗ Basilar artery
- ↗ Anterior inferior cerebellar artery
- ↗ Superior cerebellar artery
- ↗ Posterior cerebellar artery
- ↗ Spinal branches (in neck to cervical spinal cord, vertebrae and muscular branches)

43.3 Circle of Willis

To form the circle of Willis, two anterior cerebral arteries are linked by the **anterior communicating artery** (anteriorly) and posteriorly by the **posterior communicating arteries** bilaterally (Fig. 43.1). The posterior communicating arteries anastomose posteriorly with the **posterior cerebral artery**, a branch of the basilar artery.

The basilar artery is formed from the two vertebral arteries.

> ICA and ECA (and terminal CCA) can be exposed via an incision along the anterior border of SCM passing downwards from the angle of the jaw. SCM is retracted, the common facial nerve is divided, but preserving the hypoglossal nerve (crossing ECA and ICA just below the posterior digastric).
>
> To differentiate between ICA and ECA at operation: ICA is the more anterior, and gives off branches in the neck.

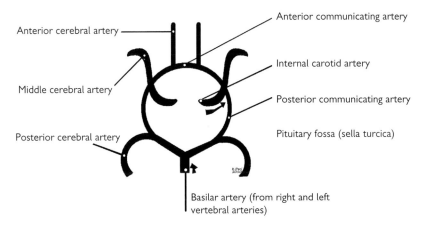

Anterior cerebral artery

Anterior communicating artery

Middle cerebral artery

Internal carotid artery

Posterior communicating artery

Posterior cerebral artery

Pituitary fossa (sella turcica)

Basilar artery (from right and left vertebral arteries)

Fig. 43.1 Circle of Willis.

43.4 Intracranial drainage

The brain has two drainage pathways:

↗ **Superficial structures** (e.g. cerebral and cerebellar cortex) drain to the nearest available **dural sinuses**

↗ **Deep structures** drain via **internal cerebral vein** on each side—formed at the **interventricular foramen** by the junction of the **choroid vein** (which drains the choroid plexus) and **thalamostriate vein**

The two cerebral veins join to form the **great cerebral vein** (the vein of Galen), which emerges from beneath the corpus callosum to meet the inferior sagittal sinus.

43.5 Dural venous sinuses

Overview

↗ The brain and skull drain into venous sinuses, which lie between the layers of the dura

↗ Ultimately drain into the IJV

↗ Also communicate with the scalp, face, and neck veins via **emissary veins**, which pass through skull foraminae

Superior sagittal sinus

↗ Lies along the attached edge of the **falx cerebri**

↗ Ends posteriorly in the **right transverse sinus**

↗ Connects with many venous lakes (**lacunae laterales**) which the **pacchionian body** of the arachnoid projects into (filtering CSF back into the blood)

Inferior sagittal sinus

↗ Lies in the free margin of the **falx cerebri**

↗ Opens into **straight sinus**

Spread of infection ± thrombosis from the lateral to sagittal sinus may impair CSF drainage into the sagittal sinus, causing hydrocephalus. If caused by an ear infection, this is known as **otitic hydrocephalus**.

Sagittal sinus thrombosis may also arrive from skull, nose, face, or scalp infections via diploic and emissary vein connections.

Straight sinus

↗ Lies in **tentorium cerebella** along the attachment of the falx cerebri

↗ Formed by the junction of **great cerebral vein** with **inferior sagittal sinus**

↗ Runs backwards to open into **left transverse sinus**

Transverse sinus

↗ Starts at internal **occipital protuberance**

↗ Runs in **tentorium cerebella** along its attached margin on either side

↗ On reaching mastoid temporal bone it forms the **sigmoid sinus**, passing inferiorly, anteriorly and medially to emerge through the jugular foramen as the IJV

Cavernous sinus

> The cavernous sinus has important relations:
>
> CN III, IV, and Va run in the lateral wall
>
> CN VI and the ICA transverses the sinus

↗ Lie either side of the sphenoid against the wall of the **pituitary fossa**

↗ Rest inferiorly on the **greater sphenoid wing**

↗ Communicate freely contralaterally via **intercavernous sinus**

↗ Traversed by **ICA, CN III, CN IV, CN V (ophthalmic and maxillary divisions)**, and **CN VI**

↗ Superiorly lie the optic tract, the uncus, and ICA

↗ Ophthalmic veins drain into the cavernous sinus, which links with the pterygoid venous plexus and anterior facial vein

↗ Receives venous drainage from the brain via superficial middle cerebral vein, and dura via sphenoparietal sinus

↗ Superior and inferior petrosal sinuses drain into the cavernous sinus and IJV respectively

Cavernous sinus infection

- Superficial infection from the face/lips/nasal sinuses can spread to the **cavernous sinus** via the anterior facial and ophthalmic veins, or deep infection via **pterygoid venous plexus** around pterygoid muscles

- Blockage of the orbital venous drainage causes conjunctival oedema and eyelids, and marked exophthalmos

- Pressure on cranial nerves produces ophthalmoplegia

- Ophthalmoscopy reveals papilloedema, venous engorgement, and retinal haemorrhages

Chapter 44 **Cranial nerves**

The cranial nerves are a favourite with examiners and you should know their main function, cranial foramina, and aspects of clinical importance.

Cranial nerves are so named as they emerge through a cranial foramen. They are part of the peripheral nervous system and the 12 pairs are named according to where they arise from the brain (anterior to posterior). They carry three major components; sensory (S), motor (M), and parasympathetic (P).

I   Olfactory nerve (S)

II   Optic nerve (S)

III   Oculomotor nerve (M, P)

IV   Trochlear nerve (M)

V   Trigeminal nerve (S, M)

       Va—ophthalmic division (S)

       Vb—maxillary division (S)

       Vc—mandibular division (S,M)

VI   Abducens nerve (M)

VII   Facial nerve (S, M, P)

VIII   Vestibulocochlear nerve (S)

IX   Glossopharyngeal nerve (S, M, P)

X   Vagus nerve (S, M, P)

XI   Accessory nerve (P)

XII   Hypoglossal nerve (P)

44.1 Olfactory nerve

⤢ Exits the cranium through the **cribiform plate** of ethmoid bone

⤢ Nerve endings (olfactory bulbs) lie on epithelial surface

⤢ Function is purely **sensory**: smell

44.2 Optic nerve

⤢ The nerve is enveloped in three layers of cerebral meninges

⤢ Cell bodies are present in the retina

⤢ The optic nerve runs through the optic canal, accompanied by the ophthalmic artery and central vein of the retina

⤢ The two optic nerves meet at the **optic chiasma**

⤢ Known as the optic tract after passing through the chiasma and terminates at the lateral geniculate body in the thalamus

⤢ Function is purely **sensory**: sight

Symptoms of optic nerve damage are dependent on site of lesion:

⤢ **Optic nerve** lesion leads to unilateral loss of sight

⤢ **Optic chiasma** lesion results in bitemporal hemianopia

⤢ **Optic tract lesion** leads to homonymous hemianopia

44.3 Oculomotor nerve

⤢ Enters the orbital cavity through the superior orbital fissure

⤢ Has both motor and parasympathetic function:

- **Motor:** Supplies superior, medial and inferior recti, inferior oblique, and levator palpebrae superior
- **Parasympathetic:** Fibres pass via the ciliary ganglion before supplying the sphincter pupillae (constricts pupil) and ciliary muscles (accommodation of lens)

⤢ Signs of an oculomotor lesion include a dilated pupil, ptosis, and a 'down and out' appearance of the eye

> Rapidly increasing intracranial pressure results in oculomotor nerve compression on the petrous part of the temporal bone. The autonomic fibres are found superficially and affected first, resulting in the earliest sign of oculomotor compression being slowed pupillary response.

44.4 Trochlear nerve

⤢ Enters the orbit through the superior orbital fissure

⤢ Function is motor and supplies the superior oblique which acts to abduct, depress, and medially rotate the eyeball

44.5 Trigeminal nerve

The trigeminal nerve consists of three branches;

Ophthalmic division (Va)

⤢ Enters the orbit via the superior orbital fissure

⤢ Function of the ophthalmic division is **sensory** to the skin of forehead, scalp, eyelids, nose, and cornea

⤢ Has five terminal branches—supraorbital, supratrochlear, lacrimal, infratrochlear, and ethmoidal nerves

Maxillary division (Vb)

⤢ Exits the cranium through the foramen rotundum

⤢ Function of maxillary division is **sensory** to the skin overlying the maxilla, upper lip, and maxillary teeth and sinus

Mandibular division (Vc)

⤢ Leaves the cranium though the foramen ovale

⤢ Has two fibre types:

- **Motor** to the muscles of mastication and also anterior belly of digastrics, mylohyoid, tensor tympani and tensor veli palatine
- **Sensory** to the skin covering the lower lip, mandible and anterior two thirds of tongue

⤢ Has four terminal branches—buccal, auriculotemporal, lingual, and inferior alveolar nerve

44.6 Abducens nerve

⤢ Enters the orbit through the superior orbital fissure

⤢ Runs close to ICA in the cavernous sinus

⤢ Function is solely **motor** to the lateral rectus which acts to move eye laterally

Commonly affected, as has a prolonged intracranial course. Patients are unable to abduct and complain of diplopia on lateral gaze.

44.7 Facial nerve

↗ Originates from the pons at the **cerebellopontine angle** and enters the middle ear through the internal auditory meatus

↗ Travels along the facial canal in the petrous portion of the temporal bone before exiting via the **stylomastoid foramen**

↗ Terminal division occurs within the parotid gland

Three important structures lie within the parotid gland (from deep):

• ECA

• Retromandibular vein

• Facial nerve

Both the nerve's path and clinical findings of a facial nerve lesion can be considered in three parts: intracranially, within the middle ear, and distal to the stylomastoid foramen.

The facial nerve has motor, sensory, and parasympathetic functions:

Motor	Supplies the muscles of facial expression, posterior belly of digastrics, stapedius, platysma, and stylohyoid
Sensory	Skin surrounding external auditory meatus and tympanic membrane, and taste from anterior two-thirds of tongue
Parasympathetic	Lacrimal, submandibular, sublingual glands

Five terminal branches of the facial nerve—**T**wo **Z**ebras **B**ashed **M**y **C**at:

↗ Temporal

↗ Zygomatic

↗ Buccal

↗ Marginal mandibular

↗ Cervical

Facial nerve has three branches in the middle ear:

↗ **Greater petrosal nerve** carries parasympathetic fibres to the lacrimal gland, and the nasal and palatine mucosa

↗ **Chorda tympani** joins and runs with the lingual nerve (branch of Vc), provides taste sensation to anterior two thirds of tongue and parasympathetic fibres to submandibular and sublingual glands

↗ **Nerve to the stapedius muscle**

Fibres of the greater petrosal nerve run via the pterygopalatine ganglion and fibres of the chorda tympani via the submandibular ganglion.

Remember: upper motor neuron lesions spare upper facial muscles. Bell's palsy is a unilateral facial paralysis: the aetiology is unknown but the facial nerve is affected in the middle ear. Distal facial nerve is commonly affected by parotid tumours or surgery.

44.8 Vestibulocochlear nerve

Function is entirely sensory, with **cochlear** and **vestibular** elements.

> An **acoustic neuroma** is a benign tumour of the Schwann cells of the vestibular nerve. Symptoms usually include hearing loss, tinnitus, and pain.

The elements initially arises together from the **cerebellopontine angle**. They enter the ear through the internal auditory meatus where they separate into:

↗ **Vestibular division** which aids balance by supplying the semicircular canals, utricle, and saccules

↗ **Cochlear division** supplies cochlea and is responsible for the sensation of hearing

44.9 Glossopharyngeal nerve

Originates from the medulla and exits the cranium through jugular foramen.

Has motor, sensory, and parasympathetic functions:

↗ Motor:
- Supplies stylopharyngeus, lifting and opening pharynx

↗ Sensory:
- Taste and sensation to posterior third of tongue
- Sensation to the palate, pharynx and carotid sinus and body

↗ Parasympathetic:
- Fibres pass through the otic ganglion supplying the parotid glands

A glossopharyngeal nerve lesion results in loss of taste to the posterior third of the tongue and loss of the gag reflex.

44.10 Vagus nerve

The vagus nerve originates from the medulla and exits through the jugular foramen. It is joined by the cranial part of accessory nerve before passing down within the carotid sheath.

The branches within the head and neck branches include pharyngeal, superior laryngeal, internal, external, and recurrent laryngeal nerves.

Has motor, sensory, and parasympathetic functions:

↗ Motor:
- Supply to pharynx, larynx, upper oesophagus, and palate

↗ Sensory:
- Skin behind auricle, pharynx, larynx, trachea, bronchi, heart, oesophagus, stomach, and intestines

↗ Parasympathetic:
- Smooth muscle of thoracic and abdominal organs

A vagus nerve lesion results in deviation of uvula to unaffected side, hoarseness of voice, and difficulty in speech and swallowing.

44.11 Accessory nerve

The accessory nerve has two roots:

Spinal root   Originating from the cervical plexus, entering the cranium through the foramen magnum and leaving through jugular foramen

Cranial root Originating from the medulla, exiting the cranium through jugular foramen before joining the vagus nerve

The spinal root has purely **motor** function and supplies the sternocleidomastoid and the trapezius.

Extracranially the spinal root is susceptible to injury in the posterior triangle of the neck where it runs on the surface of sternocleidomastoid. It runs from two-thirds of the way up the posterior border of sternocleidomastoid to one-third of the way up the anterior border of trapezius.

44.12 Hypoglossal nerve

↗ Originates from the medulla and exits the cranium through the hypoglossal canal

↗ Functions are solely **motor** as it supplies all the intrinsic and extrinsic muscles of the tongue (except palatoglossus)

A hypoglossal nerve lesion causes the tongue to deviate towards the affected side.

Chapter 45 **Cerebellum and brainstem**

45.1 Cerebellum

Located in the **infratentorial compartment**, this complex structure is concerned with posture, planning, and coordination of movement.

⤢ Consists of two hemispheres and a central **vermis**

⤢ Has numerous folds on its surface (folia) and deeper fissures dividing the cerebellar hemispheres into several lobes

The **primary fissure** separates the anterior and posterior lobes. There is a horizontal fissure within the posterior lobe; however, this does not separate the lobe and is of no functional significance.

Signs of cerebellar dysfunction—DANI

- **D**ysdiadochokinesis
- **A**taxia
- **N**ystagmus
- **I**ntention tremor

Remember: cerebellar signs are ipsilateral.

The floculonodular lobe is the most anterior and caudal part of the cerebellum consisting of the **floculus** (lateral and the nodule (the most caudal part of the vermis) This forms connections with the **vestibular system** and is functionally important for the maintenance of balance

The **cerebellar tonsil** is the most caudal part of the posterior lobe. The descent of this part of the cerebellum is associated with **Chiari malformation** and hydrocephalus.

The cerebellum is connected to the brainstem through three pairs of cerebellar peduncles:

⤢ **Superior cerebellar peduncles:**
- Connection to midbrain
- Transmit efferent fibres from cerebellum to midbrain and thalamus

⤢ **Middle cerebellar peduncles:**
- Connect the cerebellum to the pons
- Relays input from higher centres via pontine nuclei

⤢ **Inferior cerebellar peduncles:**
- Connect the cerebellum to the medulla and relay input from the vestibular nuclei, spinal cord and inferior olivary nuclei

45.2 Brainstem

⤢ Consists of the **midbrain, pons**, and **medulla**

⤢ Contains all the cranial nerve nuclei except the olfactory and optic nerves

⤢ Involved in control of eye movement; control of respiratory, cardiovascular, and autonomic function; and consciousness

⤢ Contains ascending and descending tracts

Midbrain

⤢ Cerebral peduncles found on its ventral aspect—transmit neurons from the cerebral hemispheres

⤢ Contains the cranial nerve nuclei of the **oculomotor nerve (CN III)** and **trochlear nerve (CN IV)**

⤢ The **oculomotor nerve (CN III)** emerges from the **interpeduncular fossa** between the two cerebral peduncles

↗ Structures winding round the midbrain include trochlear nerve (CN IV), optic tract, and posterior cerebral artery

↗ The **pineal gland** is located between the superior colliculi on the dorsal surface of the midbrain

↗ Pineal gland secretes melatonin which mediates the circadian rhythm

Pons

↗ Connects to cerebellum through the **middle cerebellar peduncles**

↗ Its dorsal surface forms the upper part of the floor of the IVth ventricle

↗ Cranial nerves located in the pons:

↗ **Trigeminal (CN V)** motor nucleus and part of the sensory nucleus which spans the pons and medulla)

- Abducens nerve (CN VI)
- Facial nerve (CN VII)
- Vestibulocochlear nerve (CN VIII)

↗ **Abducens nerve (CN VI)** emerges from the ventral surface at the junction between the medulla and pons

↗ Blood supply to pons is derived from pontine branches of the basilar artery

Medulla

↗ Anteriorly grooved by the anteriomedian fissure either side of which are two swelling formed by the **pyramidal tracts**

↗ Two further sulci (the anterolateral sulci) separate the pyramidal tracts from the **olivary eminences**

↗ Cranial nerves emerging from the medulla:

- Glossopharangeal nerve (CN IX)
- Vagus nerve (CN X)
- Cranial accessory nerve (CN XI)
- Hypoglossal nerve (CN XII)

↗ Connected to the cerebellum by the **inferior cerebellar peduncles**

↗ Blood supply derived directly from the **vertebral arteries** as well as from the **posterior inferior cerebellar artery branches**

The medulla contains the respiratory and cardiac centres—obviously necessary for survival. It is vulnerable to traumatic or vascular injury.

Chapter 46 **Spinal cord**

Knowledge of spinal anatomy is important for the interpretation of patterns of peripheral neurological deficit.

See Chapter 21 for anatomy of the bony vertebral column; this chapter deals with spinal cord anatomy only.

46.1 Overview

The spinal cord is continuous with the medulla at the level of the foramen magnum and tapers to the **conus medullaris** at the level of **L1/L2**. Beyond this, descending nerve roots continue as the **cauda equina.**

During early childhood, the spinal cord extends the full length of the vertebral canal. However, as a result of its differential growth compared to the vertebral column, the level of the conus 'rises' to reach its final position after the adolescent growth spurt.

The anterior surface of the cord bears a deep **anterior median fissure** extending the length of the cord.

Similarly, there is a shallow **posterior median septum** which also spans the length of the cord. Either side of this lie the **posterolateral sulci** through which the **sensory nerve roots** enter the cord.

Motor nerve roots emerge from the spinal core anterolaterally and combine with sensory nerve roots at the vertebral foramina to form the **spinal nerve** (Fig. 46.1).

> The epidural space is accessed via an interlaminar approach or via the sacral hiatus for the administration of epidural anaesthetic.

Blood supply

The spinal cord receives its blood supply from the anterior and posterior **spinal arteries** (branches of the vertebral artery).

Meninges

Like the brain, the spinal cord is encased within all three layers of meninges.

- ⤢ A continuation of the **pia mater** continues from the conus and attaches to the posterior aspect of the coccyx
- ⤢ The pia, closely adherent to the cord, has lateral thickenings (denticulate ligaments) which attach to the dura. It continues beyond the conus medullaris as the **filum terminale** which attaches to the coccyx
- ⤢ The **arachnoid mater** encloses the **subarachnoid space**, which contains CSF
- ⤢ The **dura** is single layered below the level of the foramen magnum and extends down the length of the spinal canal as far as the sacrum
- ⤢ Laterally, a sleeve of dura extends along the spinal nerve roots merging with the peripheral nerve sheath

46.2 Descending tracts

Pyramidal (lateral) corticospinal tracts

- ⤢ Commence in the cortical pyramidal cells
- ⤢ Decussate in the medulla and descend posterolaterally within the spinal cord
- ⤢ At each spinal level, fibres enter the anterior horn where they synapse with motor neurons

Anterior corticospinal tracts

- ⤢ Uncrossed fibres travelling along the wall of the anterior median fissure

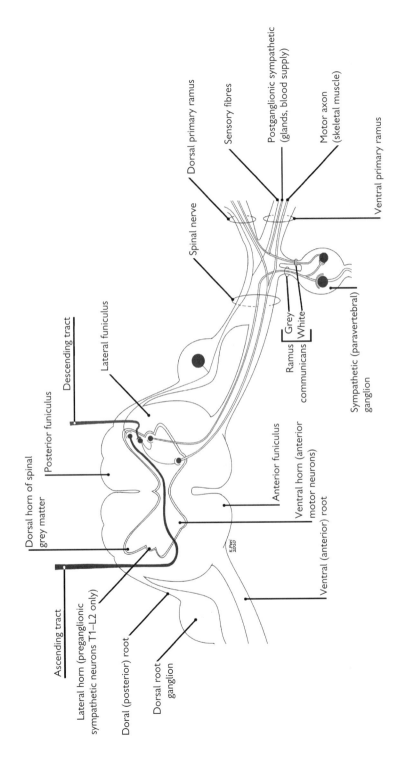

Fig 46.1 Spinal nerve root.

Postganglionic sympathetic (glands, blood supply)

Motor axon (skeletal muscle)

Dorsal primary ramus

Sensory fibres

Ventral primary ramus

Spinal nerve

Ramus communicans { Grey / White }

Sympathetic (paravertebral) ganglion

Descending tract

Lateral funiculus

Posterior funiculus

Anterior funiculus

Ventral horn (anterior motor neurons)

Dorsal horn of spinal grey matter

Ventral (anterior) root

Ascending tract

Lateral horn (preganglionic sympathetic neurons T1–L2 only)

Doral (posterior) root

Dorsal root ganglion

46.3 Ascending tracts

Dorsal columns

↗ Located between the two posterior horns of the spinal cord

↗ Consist of a medial (**fasciculus gracilis**) and a lateral (**fasciculus cuneatus**) tract

↗ Contain sensory neurons conveying light touch and proprioception

↗ Fibres remain uncrossed and synapse within the **gracile** and **cuneate nuclei** in the medulla

While some fibres travel from the medulla to the cerebellum, most of the 2nd-order neurons then decussate to the opposite thalamus where they synapse with 3rd-order neurons which travel to the sensory cortex.

Spinothalamic tracts (anterior and lateral)

↗ Contain crossed fibres transmitting pain and temperature sensation to the thalamus and then the sensory cortex

Spinocerebellar tracts

↗ Located laterally within the spinal cord and remain uncrossed until they enter the cerebellum

Cord hemisection (**Brown–Sequard syndrome**) results in:

↗ **Ipsilateral** paralysis below level (pyramidal tracts)

↗ **Iipsilateral** loss of proprioception and light touch sensation (dorsal columns)

↗ **Contralateral** loss of pain and temperature sensation (spinothalamic tracts)

Chapter 47 **Autonomic nervous system**

The autonomic nervous system controls the basic visceral and homeostatic functions of the body. Despite its importance, it is often poorly understood by candidates.

47.1 Overview

The function of the autonomic nervous system is to control of the body's internal environment. This occurs through the control of smooth muscle in the heart, gut, blood vessels, pupils, and secreto-motor functions. The autonomic nervous system is regulated by the **limbic system, hypothalamus,** and **reticular formation.** The autonomic nervous system is divided into **sympathetic** and **parasympathetic systems.**

* Unlike cranial and somatic spinal nerves, autonomic nerves synapse in peripheral ganglions close to the target organ
* The sympathetic system has its preganglionic neuron cell bodies within the **lateral horns** of the thoracolumbar spinal cord **(T1–L3)**
* The parasympathetic system has its preganglionic neuronal cell bodies within the **brainstem** and **sacral plexus**

47.2 Sympathetic nervous system

The sympathetic nervous system is concerned mainly with the body's response to stress. Its postsynaptic neurotransmitter in most cases is adrenaline and noradrenaline (except for sympathetic supply to sweat glands in which the neurotransmitter is acetylcholine). Sympathetic efferent fibres leave their origin in the lateral horns of T1–L3 via the **ventral primary rami.** These then travel to the sympathetic chain via **white rami communicans**

Actions

* Papillary dilatation
* Increase of heart rate
* Dilatation of respiratory smooth muscle

Sympathetic chain

* Located either side of the vertebral column and extends the full length of the spine
* Passes into the abdomen via the **arcuate ligament** of the diaphragm
* Descends between psoas muscle and the lumbar vertebrae
* Enters the pelvis and terminates at the **ganglion impar** over the coccyx

47.3 Parasympathetic nervous system

* Has cranial and sacral components
* Preganglionic fibres synapse with ganglion cells close to or within the target organ

Cranial component

* Conveyed in cranial nerves III, VII, IX, and X
* Actions:

Papillary constriction	CN III
Lacrimation and salivation	CN VII and CN IX
Slowing heart rate	CN X
Slowing of bowel function and bronchoconstriction	CN X

Sacral component

↗ Derived from fibres arising from S2, 3, and 4

↗ Joins the **pudendal plexus** before being distributed to pelvic organs

↗ Termed the 'nerves of emptying', the sacral parasympathetic system supplies **visceromotor** input to the rectum and bladder wall, as well as inhibitory supply to the internal anal sphincter and internal vesical sphincters

↗ Has a **vasodilatory effect** on the cavernous sinuses of the penis and clitoris

Process of micturition

• Cerebral removal of conscious inhibition

• Waves of detrusor muscle contraction and relaxation of internal and external sphincters (**parasympathetic**)

• On completion of voiding—relaxation of detrusor muscle, contraction of internal sphincter (**sympathetic**) and external sphincters (**voluntary**)

Section 2 Pathology and Physiology

Chapter 48 **Cerebrospinal fluid: formation and flow**

The production, constituents, and flow of cerebrospinal fluid (CSF) are fundamental to neurosurgery. Candidates for the MRCS examination must be familiar not only with the physiology and anatomy of CSF, but also common procedures of shunts and diversions.

48.1 Cerebrospinal fluid

The CSF is clear fluid which occupies the subarachnoid space, ventricular system, and around the spinal cord and nerve roots as well as the central canal of spinal cord. An adult has approximately 150 mL of CSF evenly distributed intracranially and spinally.

Functions

- Mechanical shock absorption
- Suspension of brain (i.e. brain 'floats' in CSF, preventing crushing of lower portion of the brain under its own weight)
- Biochemical homeostasis
- Haemodynamic homeostasis

> Biochemical homeostasis involves regulation of pH and glucose as well circulating hormones and immune factors.

Production

- At a rate of 500 mL daily (equivalent to full turnover thrice daily)
- Mainly in choroid plexus but also in walls of lateral, IIIrd and IVth ventricles, and spinal cord

Absorption

- Arachnoid villi (protrude into the dural venous sinuses)

Flow

After production mainly in the choroid plexus the CSF follows the following path (Fig. 48.1, Fig. 48.2):

- Lateral ventricles
- Through foramen of Monro
- IIIrd ventricle
- Aqueduct of Sylvius
- IVth ventricle
- Foramina of Magendie and Luschka
- Subarachnoid space around brain and spinal cord

Constituents

See Table 48.1.

48.2 Hydrocephalus

Hydrocephalus is the abnormal accumulation of CSF within the ventricular system. Often but not always associated with a dilatation of the ventricular system and rise in intracranial pressure (ICP).

Classification

- Overproduction (e.g. the very rare choroid plexus papilloma) or more commonly an abnormality of CSF circulation or absorption
- Speed of onset (i.e. acute or chronic)
- Aetiology (communicating or noncommunicating)

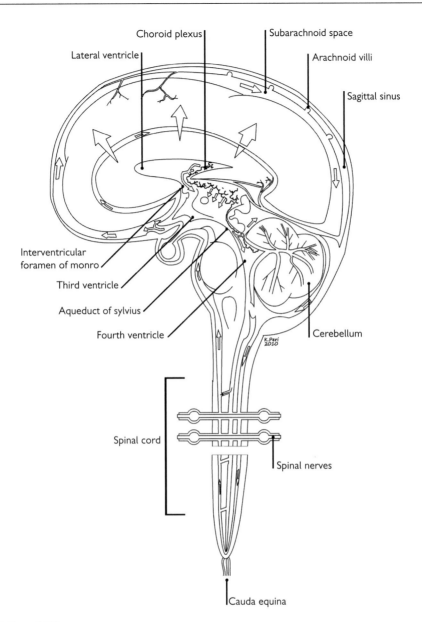

Fig. 48.1 Flow of CSF.

Causes

Communicating

↗ Congenital:

- Arnold Chiari malformation
- Encephalocele

↗ Acquired:

- Normal pressure hydrocephalus (60% no known aetiology)

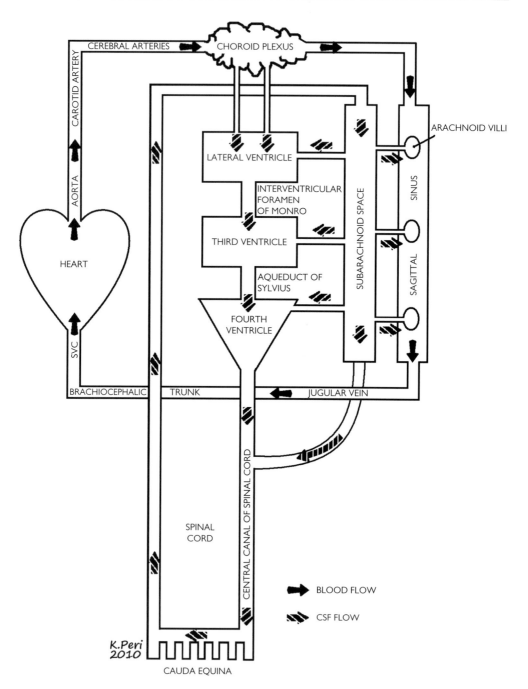

Fig. 48.2 Diagram of CSF production and flow.

Table 48.1 Constituents of CSF

	CSF content	Plasma content
Na^{2+}	138 mEq L^{-1}	138 mEq L^{-1}
K^+	2.8 mEq L^{-1}	4.5 mEq L^{-1}
Cl$^-$	119 mEq L^{-1}	102 mEq L^{-1}
Ca^{2+}	2.1 mEq L^{-1}	4.8 mEq L^{-1}
Glucose	60 mL dL^{-1}	90 mL dL^{-1}
Total protein	35 mg dL^{-1}	7000 mL dL^{-1}

- Infective (e.g. post meningitis)
- Haemorrhage—subarachnoid haemorrhage (SAH) or intraventricular haemorrhage (IVH) in infancy
- Venous hypertension (e.g. sinus thrombosis)
- Leptomeningeal
- Carcinomatosis
- CSF-producing tumours (e.g. choroid plexus papilloma)
- Hydrocephalus *ex vacuo* (e.g. post infarction)

Noncommunicating

↗ Congenital:

- Aqueduct stenosis
- Dandy Walker malformation (atresia of foramen of Luschka and Magendi)
- Vascular malformation

↗ Acquired:

- Tumours (e.g. IIIrd ventricular, posterior fossa, pineal region)
- Ventricular scarring

Remember: when asked for 'causes of...', **never** just start listing causes, but always open with 'Causes of hydrocephalus are divided into communicating and noncommunicating ...'

Clinical presentation

Neonates

↗ Bulging fontanelles

↗ Prominent scalp veins

↗ 'Sunsetting' eyes due to CSF pressure on the midbrain tectum

↗ Papilloedema

↗ Disproportionate head growth (measured by the occipitofrontal head circumference and plotted on a centile chart)

↗ Irritability, poor feeding, slow to reach developmental milestones

Adults

↗ Symptoms of raised ICP: headaches, nausea, vomiting, drowsiness, papilloedema and blurred vision

↗ Loss of upward gaze

⤴ Cognitive impairment, poor concentration, and behavioural changes may be sign of hydrocephalus of insidious onset

⤴ Normal pressure hydrocephalus has a characteristic clinical triad of:

- Gait disturbance
- Urinary incontinence
- Dementia

In any age group, a loss of consciousness with associated bradycardia, hypertension, and abnormal respiration may signal critical life-threatening hydrocephalus and requires prompt treatment.

Investigation

Cranial ultrasound scanning

This is a noninvasive and readily available tool, often used for the age group where fontanelles are open, to monitor ventricular size and identify causes—e.g. intraventricular haemorrhage, intraventricular tumours.

Head CT and MRI

Ventricular size alone is an unreliable in the diagnosis of hydrocephalus on a CT or MRI scan. Additional features on CT/MRI suggestive of hydrocephalus include:

⤴ Periventricular oedema

⤴ Enlargement of the temporal horns (>2 mm), lateral ventricles, and IIIrd ventricle

⤴ Obliteration of cortical sulci and gyri and effacement of basal cisterns

48.3 Management of hydrocephalus

CSF external drainage

Lumbar puncture and lumbar drains

⤴ Frequently used as a temporary CSF drainage measure until or normal circulation/resorption resumes

⤴ Should only be considered in communicating hydrocephalus where an intracranial mass lesion has been ruled out on head CT or MRI

⤴ Great care should be taken not to overdrain as this can give rise to subdural haemorrhage or cerebellar tonsillar herniation

External ventricular drainage (EVD)

⤴ Often used in the acute setting (e.g. SAH) where hydrocephalus may be transient and a permanent shunt can sometimes be avoided

⤴ May be used as a temporizing measure where the high particulate content of CSF (e.g. protein in postmeningitic hydrocephalus or RBCs in IVH) make the risk of early shunt blockage high

⤴ Can be used to administer intrathecal medication in for the treatment of ventriculitis

Permanent shunts

Ventriculo-peritoneal (VP) shunt

⤴ Commonest shunt procedure

⤴ Proximal catheter inserted into lateral ventricle connected to distal catheter which is tunnelled subcutaneously to the abdomen where it is inserted into the peritoneal cavity where the CSF is absorbed

↗ There is a wide variety of shunt valves designed to provide different CSF flow or pressure rates depending on the clinical condition

↗ When an obstruction occurs at the level of the foramen of Munroe, bilateral VP shunts may be inserted

↗ Complications include obstruction, infection, breakage/erosion, seizures, or abdominal complications

Ventriculo-atrial (VA) shunt

↗ Shunt of choice where abdominal abnormalities (e.g. extensive abdominal surgery, peritonitis, morbid obesity) preclude the insertion of a VP shunt

↗ Distal catheter is inserted via the jugular vein to the superior vena cava

↗ Complications include infection/septicaemia, shunt embolism, short catheter length (requires repeated lengthening in a growing child), perforation, pulmonary hypertension

Lumbo-peritoneal (LP) shunt

↗ Only used in communicating hydrocephalus

↗ Complications include progressive cerebellar tonsillar descent, lumbar radiculopathy due to nerve root irritation, overshunting, adhesions, arachnoiditis

Medical treatment

Appropriate in certain circumstances:

↗ Osmotic diuretics such as mannitol may be used as a temporizing measure in the acute situation (e.g. blocked shunt)

↗ Where a transient reduction in ICP is required pending definitive surgical treatment

↗ Acetazolamide is a carbonic anhydrase inhibitor which inhibits CSF production. It is often used in benign intracranial hypertension in neonates as a temporizing measure while the child gains weight prior to a shunt procedure

Chapter 49 Intracranial homeostasis and head injury

A large amount of a neurosurgeon's workload is management of head injuries. An understanding of neurophysiology means surgeons often don't have to perform any surgery at all!

49.1 Background

A neurosurgeon is referred many different types of head injury. This can be stratified by mechanism, severity, or morphology

Specifics of trauma and intracranial lesions are covered in other chapters; here we will encourage the candidate to think about neurophysiology and homeostasis.

Neurons that are injured have the ability to either recover or die. Much of the work of the neurosurgeon is creating optimum conditions to allow prevalence of the former.

First principles

In any line of questioning, never forget to discuss the relevance of ABC/ATLS™ in the initial approach to head injury.

Airway compromise can kill head-injured patients before they even reach hospital. Patients often have associated injuries, and many patients turn up to the Emergency Department hypotensive and hypoxic. These all must be corrected before assessing head injury, as if this is not done correctly outcome is seriously affected.

Glasgow Coma Scale

The Glasgow Coma Scale (GCS), devised by Teasdale and Jennett in 1974 at Glasgow's Institute of Neurological Sciences, breaks down conscious levels to eye opening, verbalization, and obeying commands.

Mechanism
- ↗ Closed RTA, falls, blunt trauma
- ↗ Open Missile injury

Severity
- ↗ Mild GCS 14–15
- ↗ Moderate GCS 9–13
- ↗ Severe GCS 3–8

Think
- ↗ Apnoea
- ↗ Aspiration
- ↗ Atelectasis

CT scan indications
- ↗ Loss of consciousness
- ↗ Amnesia
- ↗ Vague history
- ↗ Significant mechanism
- ↗ Signs of skull fractures
- ↗ Headache, nausea and vomiting
- ↗ Seizures
- ↗ Neurological deficit

Abnormal images should ideally be reported by a radiologist before being referred to a neurosurgeon (neurosurgeons are good at reading scans but are not radiologists; having a formal opinion can make referring patients easier). All patients with confirmed head injury should ideally be observed in a centre specializing in neurosurgery, but the absence of this should not prevent patients being admitted or transferred appropriately and safely.

49.2 Intracranial homeostasis

Blood–brain barrier

↗ Often disrupted in head injury

↗ The principle of the blood–brain barrier is tight junctions (known as **zona occludens**) between endothelial cells of the cerebral capillaries

↗ Disruption of the blood–brain barrier will cause leakage of blood and vasogenic oedema

Intracranial pressure

Measured in mmHg; normally 10–15 mmHg

Monroe–Kellie hypothesis

This is based on the theory that the skull is an enclosed box: the sum of the intracranial constituents is constant, therefore an increase in one of the constituents results in a decrease in another. If this doesn't happen then ICP will increase

Cerebral perfusion pressure

This is a very important measurement in the injured brain. It is calculated as

CPP = MAP – ICP

where CPP is the cerebral perfusion pressure, MAP is the mean arterial pressure, and ICP is the intracranial pressure.

This partly explains the importance of ABC/ATLS™ in head injury management, as hypotensive head injury patients are clearly less likely to perfuse the brain adequately.

> In injured brain, CPP is often kept above 70 mmHg.

Autoregulation

↗ Normally blood will flow to active parts of the brain

↗ The brain is able to regulate adequate perfusion at a cerebral perfusion pressure of 50–150 mmHg via vasoconstriction of cerebral arterioles

↗ Blood pressures outside this range can adversely affect cerebral perfusion

> Head injury disrupts cerebral autoregulation.

49.3 Management

The previous section emphasizes that neuronal survival is dependent on delivery of oxygenated blood to the brain and maintaining a normal ICP.

Common day-to-day management of head injury patients is tailored towards controlling ICP.

> Aim for pCO_2 4.0–4.5 kPa. Think:
>
> ↗ Pyrexia
>
> ↗ Seizures
>
> ↗ Infection

⤤ Light sedation

⤤ Electrolyte abnormalities

⤤ Hypercapnia

Correcting all of the above must always be the first priority in the head-injured patient. This must be done in conjunction with the intensivist who can adjust ventilator settings accordingly, and adjust sedation in patients who may be inadequately sedated.

Remember: in head injury:

⤤ Tilt bed to 'head up 30°'

⤤ Can collars be removed?

It is important to consider that any seizures may not be clinically obvious, particularly in ventilated patients, so an EEG is worth considering. In cases of altered neurology, repeat imaging is always important to exclude surgical cause.

Most consultants will favour anticonvulsants in head-injured patients. Also, all patients where ICP is expected to rise (e.g. intracerebral contusions) should be considered for ICP monitoring.

When the above abnormalities have been considered, final steps are chemical coma with barbiturates such as phenobarbital, which decrease cerebral metabolism.

People will often suggest mannitol (an osmotic diuretic), when in fact it is one of the later options in management of ICP. It should be given IV at 200 mL of 20% mannitol. It is commonly used to 'buy time' before transfer to CT scan or to a specialist centre for definitive management. Repeated usage renders it ineffectual (keep serum osmolality <320 mmol/kg).

Surgery

Surgical emergencies resulting in raised ICP (e.g. extradural haematoma, intracerebral haematoma) ought to be decompressed as a surgical emergency.

Recalling the Monroe–Kellie doctrine, procedures such as EVD can divert CSF from the intracranial cavity to an external bag, creating extra space within the cranium.

The final surgical step is the decompressive craniectomy, where a portion of the skull is removed and the dura mater opened, allowing the brain to expand outwards.

Senior decision-making is crucial in these cases, as it may well be futile to continue treatment.

Chapter 50 **Central nervous system infections**

CNS infections can be rapidly progressive and life-threatening. Early diagnosis and institution of medical therapy and or surgical intervention is essential.

50.1 Meningitis

Causes of bacterial meningitis
- ↗ Direct transmission from nearby infected structures (e.g. nasopharyngeal infection, osteomyelitis)
- ↗ Penetrating wound (e.g. open skull fracture)
- ↗ Blood-borne infection resulting from septicaemia
- ↗ Iatrogenic (e.g. postsurgical meningitis)

Common causative organism

Neonates	*Haemophilus influenzae* (type B), Gram −ve bacilli (e.g. *E. coli*)
Children	*H. influenzae*, *Streptococcus pneumoniae*, meningococci
Adults	*S. pneumoniae*, meningococci

Clinical features
- ↗ Commonly presents with the triad of:
  - Headache
  - Fever
  - Neck stiffness
- ↗ Meningism
- ↗ Impaired GCS
- ↗ Cranial nerve deficit
- ↗ Focal neurological deficit (limb paresis, visual and speech problems)

> Positive **Kernig's sign**—stretching of lumbar nerve roots by flexing the hip and extending the knee produces marked discomfort.

Investigation
- ↗ CT head, to exclude and intracranial mass, haemorrhage, or hydrocephalus, especially if the patient has a reduced GCS
- ↗ Lumbar puncture, only once CT head has excluded any intracranial mass lesion
- ↗ Measurement of CSF pressure prior to sending a sample microscopy, culture and sensitivity
- ↗ Blood cultures
- ↗ Septic screen to investigate possible causes

Treatment
- ↗ Antibiotic treatment should be commenced as soon as diagnosis is suspected. Do not delay to identify causative organism!
- ↗ Initial therapy—benzylpenicillin (cefotaxime if penicillin allergic)
- ↗ Consider additional steroid therapy starting with the first dose of antibiotics
- ↗ Complications include; epilepsy, cerebral abscess or subdural empyema, cerebral infarction

50.2 Cerebral abscess

- ↗ Usually forms as a consequence of chronic or persistent cerebral infection
- ↗ Origins of infection are similar to those causing meningitis:
  - Direct spread from adjacent infected structures (e.g. sinusitis, blood-borne, or as a consequence of penetrating injury)

⤢ Can cause rapid clinical deterioration and should be diagnosed and treated quickly

⤢ Lumbar puncture should **not** be performed. Cerebral abscesses are associated with significant brain swelling and raised ICP

⤢ Once diagnosed, treatment requires antibiotic therapy, steroids, and consideration of early surgical drainage to establish causative organism and relief of intracranial mass effect

Chapter 51 **Central nervous system tumours**

51.1 Overview

Epidemiology

↗ The annual incidence of newly diagnosed brain tumours in the UK is 4500

↗ Accounts for 2% of all cancers and 2% of all cancer deaths

↗ The overall mortality rate from brain and other CNS tumours in the UK is 4000/year

↗ The most common intracranial neoplasm in adults is metastases, accounting for just under 50%, followed by gliomas (25%)

Classification

↗ Metastases

↗ Primary intrinsic neoplasm

↗ Extrinsic neoplasm

Presentation

↗ Features of raised ICP: headaches, nausea ± vomiting, papilloedema

↗ Mental status change/reduction in GCS

↗ Seizures

↗ Focal neurological deficit (cranial nerve palsy or motor deficit)

Investigation

↗ CT head:

• Single or multiple lesions of variable size with associated oedema

• Often show enhancement with contrast

↗ MRI brain:

• More sensitive than CT at identifying small or multiple metastatic lesions

• Investigation of the primary lesion

Management

↗ Corticosteroids:

• Reduction of oedema associated with intracranial metastases gives temporary clinical improvement

↗ Biopsy:

• Informs further investigation of the primary and overall treatment

↗ Resection:

• May be undertaken for single intracranial metastases where accessible

↗ Stereotactic radiosurgery:

↗ Useful alternative to surgery for smaller lesions (<3 cm) or those inaccessible for surgical resection

> Metastases are the most common intracranial neoplasms in adults, and questions on source primary neoplasms are very common question in examinations.

51.2 Intracranial metastases

Primary lesions

Lung	40%
Breast	19%

Melanoma	10%
Genitourinary	7%
Female genital	5%
Gastrointestinal	7%

Features

⤢ Spread is usually haematogenous to the grey/white matter junction

- The venous route is also possible via a pelvic–vertebral venous plexus (Batson's plexus) to the posterior fossa
- 25% of intracranial metastases are to the posterior fossa
- Bony intracranial metastases most commonly arise from a prostate and breast primary
- Metastases into the sella turcica most commonly arise from a breast primary
- Cerebral metastases are often multiple

51.3 Primary intrinsic tumours

These arise from within the brain substance.

Classification

Modern classification system is the WHO classification, based on cell type and degree of anaplasia:

Grade I	Pliocytic astrocytoma
Grade II	Astrocytoma
Grade III	Anaplastic astrocytoma
Grade IV	Glioblastoma multiforme

Low grade (I–II)

⤢ Account for approximately 15% of all primary intracranial tumours

⤢ Diffuse, slow growing

⤢ Subdivided into fibrillary, protoplasmic, and gemistocytic types

⤢ Up to 90 % show loss of p53

⤢ Pilocytic types occur in children and young adults

⤢ Common sites include hypothalamic area, optic nerve (in association with NF-1), cerebellum and brainstem

CT/MRI features

⤢ May be difficult to identify especially at early stages

⤢ An area of low density on CT with or without enhancement

⤢ MRI may demonstrate low intensity lesion on T1-weighted image which may or may not enhance with gadolinium

⤢ T2-weighted image may better demonstrate lesion and surrounding oedema

Management

⤢ Corticosteroids

⤢ Biopsy

⤢ Surgical craniotomy

Prognosis

- Resection can be curative
- 5-year survival for grade II astrocytoma is 50–60%
- Grade I pilocytic astrocytoma show up to 80% 20-year survival

High grade (III–IV)

- Rapidly growing with high malignancy
- Account for 40% of intracranial tumours in adults
- Peak incidence at 40–50s
- Very poor prognosis
- Two types of glioblastoma:
  - Primary glioblastoma—arise de-novo
  - Secondary glioblastoma—dedifferentiate from lower-grade intrinsic tumours

CT/MRI features

- Space-occupying lesion of mixed density/intensity
- Irregular contrast enhancement
- Often central low density/intensity and surrounding oedema
- Often causes mass effect as seen by effacement of ventricles, sulci, and gyri as well as a shift of the midline

Management

- Corticosteroids
- Biopsy
- Surgical debulking
- Radiotherapy
- Chemotherapy:
  - Agents used include nitrosoureas and temozolamide
  - Intraoperative insertion of carmustine-impregnated wafers into the tumour bed has also been show to improve survival

Prognosis

- Mean survival for untreated high-grade glioma is 3–4 months
- This is improved to 6 months with surgical debulking alone and 9–10 months with debulking and adjuvant radiotherapy

51.4 Extrinsic tumours

Three main types: meningioma, pituitary tumour, and vestibular schwannoma

Meningioma

- Slow-growing, benign tumour arising from the arachnoid granulations
- Constitute 20% of all primary intracranial tumours
- Commonest age group is 40–60 years
- Usually benign tumour but sometimes undergoes malignant change (1–2%)
- Causes reactive hyperostosis and may invade adjacent bone

Presentation

↗ Epilepsy

↗ Symptoms of raised intracranial pressure

↗ Focal neurological deficit (depending on tumour location)

↗ Visual disturbances or visual field defects (especially with medial sphenoid wing meningiomas)

↗ Cranial nerve palsies

Investigation

Skull radiograph	Bony hyperostosis with radiating spicules (sunray effect) and calcification seen in 15%
CT	Well-demarcated, homogenous, isodense or hyperdense lesion which may be calcified or with surrounding oedema
MRI	Isointense on T1-weighted image; striking enhancement with IV gadolinium contrast
Angiography	Useful to identify these characteristically very vascular lesions and if possible embolize feeding vessels preoperatively

Management

↗ Corticosteroids

↗ Antiepileptics—particularly useful preoperatively

↗ Surgical resection is undertaken with the aim of complete resection of the tumour and its meningeal origin

  • Recurrence depends on the completeness of tumour resection: 20% will recur after 10 years following complete macroscopic resection while 50% recur following subtotal resection

Pituitary tumour

↗ Constitute 5–10% of intracranial tumours

↗ Usually benign and arise from the anterior pituitary

Classification

↗ Clinical classification subdivides pituitary tumours into **microadenomas** (tumour size <1 cm) and **macroadenomas** (>1 cm)

↗ Also classified on basis of hormone secreted by tumour:

Prolactinoma	25–50%
Nonfunctioning adenoma	25–40%
GH-secreting tumours	20–25%
ACTH-secreting tumours	5–10%
TSH- and FSH/LH- secreting tumours	Very rare

Clinical presentation

Due to local mass effect or endocrine dysfunction.

↗ Local mass effect:

  • Headache

  • Visual field defect, commonly bitemporal hemianopia

↗ Endocrine dysfunction:

  • Prolactinoma—commonest type of pituitary tumour causing menstrual dysfunction in women and infertility or impotence in men

  • GH-secreting tumour—results in acromegaly when it occurs in adults, or gigantism when it occurs in children where epiphyses are yet to fuse

Signs of acromegaly
- Enlarged face, hands, and feet
- Coarse skin
- Hyperhydrosis
- Hypertension
- Diabetes (10%)

- ACTH-secreting tumour—stimulates secretion of cortisol and androgens from the adrenal glands

Cushing's syndrome
- Causes:
  - Pituitary adenoma (Cushing's disease)
  - Bilateral adrenal hyperplasia
  - Excessive exogenous steroid administration
  - Adrenal tumour
  - ACTH-secreting bronchial carcinoma, medullary thyroid carcinoma or carcinoid tumour
- Clinical features:
  - Face—moon face, acne, baldness + hirsutism
  - Trunk—central obesity, buffalo hump, abdominal striae, muscle weakness, bruising
  - Systemic—hypertension, diabetes mellitus, osteoporosis, increased infections

Remember: an ACTH-secreting pituitary adenoma is Cushing's **disease**, but one cause of Cushing's **syndrome**

Management

Medical
- Dopamine agonists (e.g. cabergoline or bromocriptine) used to reduce hormone levels, especially prolactin, which often shrinks tumour

Surgical management
- Transsphenoidal resection
- Transcranial surgery

Radiotherapy
- Most pituitary tumours are radiosensitive

Vestibular schwannoma

Also referred to as **acoustic neuroma**. These are benign lesions arising from the vestibular portion of the VIIIth nerve.
- Constitute 6% of primary intracranial tumours
- Usually present around the 5th decade of life
- Bilateral vestibular schwannoma are associated with neurofibromatosis type II
- Located in the cerebellopontine angle

Clinical features

➢ Slowly progressive, often unilateral sensorineural deafness

➢ Vertigo and tinnitus are rare features, because of the slow pace of tumour growth which allows for compensation

➢ Compression of neighbouring cranial nerves

Management

➢ Conservative approach:

• Small tumours not causing symptoms may be observed with serial imaging

➢ Surgical excision:

• Several approaches, the aim of which is to achieve maximal tumour resection with preservation of facial nerve function and hearing if not already lost

Section 3 **Clinical**

Chapter 52 **Neuroradiology**

The MRCS does not require candidates to become experts in radiology; however, an understanding of the radiological appearance of common conditions and appropriate use of current/future imaging will reflect well on any candidate.

52.1 Presenting scans

This may sound obvious, but so many marks are available for talking in a structured and knowledgeable way.

↗ Is it a CT or an MRI?

↗ What is the weighting (T1/T2) and is contrast used?

↗ What plane is the scan?

> **Planes**
>
> ↗ Axial (transverse)
>
> ↗ Sagittal
>
> ↗ Coronal

This simple structure will show the examiner that you have a good level of basic knowledge. It is then advisable to work through the scan in a structured fashion, before diving straight to the obvious abnormality. For example, a candidate could describe accurately the presence of subarachnoid blood, yet miss the early appearance of hydrocephalus which could be clinically significant.

> **Look at this scan and tell me what you think**
>
> 'This is an axial CT scan of the brain taken without contrast. Starting from the skull base moving towards the vertex the scan shows that the basal cisterns are open, although there is mild enlargement of the temporal horns. Around the circle of Willis there is diffuse hyperdensity in the subarachnoid space. Continuing towards the vertex there is no evidence of mass effect or cerebral oedema. In my opinion the scan is consistent with subarachnoid haemorrhage with early hydrocephalus.'

In the lead-up to the examination, get into the habit of mentally going through this structure in your head when looking at an example. Avoid looking at the report until you have gone through the scan yourself, then compare your findings with the radiologist's report. You may be surprised just how much you begin to pick up with practice.

> **Remember:**
>
> ↗ CT scans display **density**
>
> ↗ MRI scans display **intensity**

52.2 Stroke and head injury

Normal anatomy and imaging modalities

Any understanding of neuroradiology requires knowledge of the circle of Willis, which supplies the arterial blood supply to the brain. Although this has been covered in detail earlier, in the context of radiology try thinking about the circle of Willis in the following way:

↗ It is broadly divided into the **anterior** and **posterior** circulations, with the anterior arising from the carotid arteries and the posterior from the vertebral arteries

↗ The anterior and posterior circulations are linked by the **posterior communicating artery**; however, this artery is normally only partially filled, only diverting flow when there is resistance to flow in one of the circulations

Radiologists often separate the **anterior** cerebral and **middle** cerebral arteries into segments termed **A1, A2**, and **M1, M2** respectively. This is normally between the branches; for example M1 is the segment

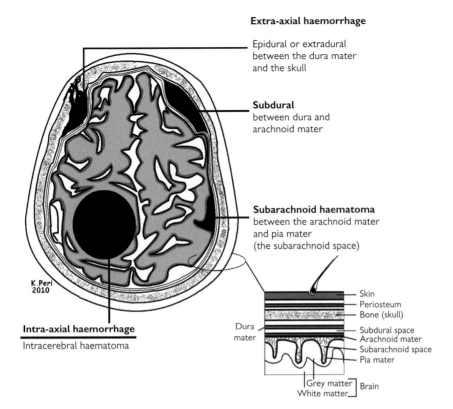

Extra-axial haemorrhage

Epidural or extradural
between the dura mater
and the skull

Subdural
between dura and
arachnoid mater

Subarachnoid haematoma
between the arachnoid mater
and pia mater
(the subarachnoid space)

Skin
Periosteum
Bone (skull)
Dura mater
Subdural space
Arachnoid mater
Subarachnoid space
Pia mater

Grey matter ⎤ Brain
White matter ⎦

K.Peri
2010

Intra-axial haemorrhage
Intracerebral haematoma

Fig. 52.1 Classification of intracranial bleeds.

of the middle cerebral artery between its origin at the internal carotid and the first branch. Using this terminology can make you sound particularly knowledgeable when describing the location of a vascular lesion such as an aneurysm.

A classification of cranial bleeding is shown in Fig 52.1.

Subdural haematoma

* Crescentic
* Can cross sutures (except sagittal)
* Does not cross the tentorium
* Flattens the sulci
* Mass effect

Subdurals on CT

* Acute (<1 week)—hyperdense
* Subacute (1–3 weeks)—isodense
* Chronic (>3 weeks)—hypodense
* Central, swirling 'lucency'—active bleeding

Extradural haematoma

- ↗ Coup lesions
- ↗ Do **not** cross sutures
- ↗ Can cross the tentorium
- ↗ Often underlying fractures
- ↗ May be contrecoup subdural
- ↗ Midline shift

Haemorrhagic contusions

- ↗ Early CT—normal appearance or hypodensity
- ↗ 24–48 hours—new lesions, enlarged lesions
- ↗ Reach maximum swelling over 5–7 days

Diffuse axonal injury

- ↗ MRI better than CT
  - ◆ CT often initially normal
- ↗ Petechial haemorrhages, hypodensities on CT
- ↗ Poor prognosis

> **Diffuse axonal injury**
> - ↗ Caused by shearing motion of axons
> - ↗ Poor prognosis

Infarction

- ↗ Wedge-shaped hypodensity on CT
- ↗ Ischaemic 'penumbra'
- ↗ Dense middle cerebral artery infarction may have 'ribbon sign'
- ↗ Beware infarcts producing oedema and mass effect

52.3 Spinal radiology

The most likely subject to be presented in the examination is cervical spine trauma, but degenerative processes may also come up.

Cervical spine

Cervical spine series (for trauma)

- ↗ AP view
- ↗ Peg view
- ↗ Lateral view
- ↗ Alignment
- ↗ Prevertebral soft tissues
- ↗ Other bones (skull base)

NB: a swimmer's or oblique view may be necessary for the lateral view to be adequate—C1 to superior border of T1.

Atlanto-occipital dislocation

⤢ Highly unstable injury

⤢ Frequent associated neurological injury

⤢ Common rupture of the tectorial membrane

⤢ Rupture of alar ligaments

⤢ Often occipital condyle fractures

Atlas fractures

⤢ Isolated posterior arch fractures are stable

⤢ Jefferson (burst) fractures due to axial loading are unstable

Odontoid peg (dens) fractures

Type 1   Oblique fracture through the upper part of the peg; these are stable injuries

Type 2   Fracture through base of peg; unstable injury with nonunion a common complication

Type 3   Involves body of axis, unstable but usually unite

Cervical spine flexion injuries

⤢ Anterior subluxation

⤢ Bilateral facet dislocation

⤢ Wedge fractures (see below)

Three-column theory of spinal fractures

⤢ Column 1—anterior half of body

⤢ Column 2—posterior body to facets

⤢ Column 3—posterior elements

Fractures of two or more columns are **unstable.**

Degenerative disease and compressive spinal pathology

Classification of spinal lesions

Extradural	Outside the thecal sac (includes bone)
Intradural	• Also called extramedullary
	• Within the theca but outside the cord
Intramedullary	Within the cord

Common extradural lesions

⤢ Herniated disc

⤢ Vertebral haemangioma

⤢ Bony metastases

⤢ Epidural abscess

⤢ Synovial cyst

Common intradural/extramedullary lesions

⤢ Meningioma

⤢ Metastases

⤢ Nerve sheath tumour (e.g. schwannoma)

Chapter 53 **Common neurosurgical cases**

53.1 Background

The MRCS syllabus identifies core topics for examination:

⤢ Head injuries

⤢ Intracranial haemorrhage

  ◆ Subarachnoid

  ◆ Intracerebral

  ◆ Subdural

  ◆ Extradural

  ◆ Intraventricular

⤢ Brain injuries

⤢ Spinal cord injuries

⤢ Assessment and resuscitation of the comatose patient

⤢ Paralytic disorders

⤢ Peripheral nerve injuries

Specifically, at this level candidates should confidently understand the clinical presentation of trauma, intracranial masses, and tumours of the central and peripheral nervous system.

Here we present cases that broadly cover all of the above topics and the most likely question avenues.

53.2 Subarachnoid haemorrhage

History

⤢ Sudden severe headache

⤢ No trauma

⤢ Altered conscious level

Examination

Inspect Fundoscopy

Test • GCS
     • Photophobia
     • Neck stiffness
     • Neurological examination

Present

'This 41-year old woman presents with severe headache, photophobia, and a painful neck. Vital signs are stable. Her eyes are open and she obeys commands but thinks she is still in her living room at home. There are no focal neurological deficits.'

Likely questions

1. Discuss the causes of this condition

Overall, the most common cause is trauma. In cases of spontaneous subarachnoid haemorrhage (SAH) an **aneurysmal bleed** is the most common culprit—most commonly from the circle of Willis, although giant aneurysms from the internal carotid are sometimes seen. Further causes are **arteriovenous malformations** (AVMs), and bleeding into tumours. Occasionally blood is located purely around the midbrain and no vascular abnormality is found—these are known as **paramesencephalic SAHs** and are of uncertain origin.

Causes of spontaneous SAH

⤢ Aneurysms

⤢ AVM

⤢ Tumour bleed

⤢ Unknown

2. Describe the likely investigations in this case

Patients being admitted must have routine haematological investigations, specifically clotting studies. A patient with this presentation needs a CT scan of the head, and if blood is seen a **CT angiogram** can be performed to assess the cerebral vasculature. If no vascular abnormality is seen, the case ought to be discussed with a neuroradiologist to advise whether to proceed with a formal catheter digital subtraction angiogram (DSA). This investigation has the advantage of allowing immediate treatment of most aneurysms via endovascular platinum helical coiling.

If CT scanning is negative and clinical suspicion prevails, the next investigation would be a lumbar puncture. The main purpose of the test is to show RBC within the CSF (although be wary of traumatic sampling). If the presentation is >12 hours after onset of symptoms it is worth sending a sample for **xanthochromia**. This is due to breakdown products of haemoglobin in the CSF, and has the advantage of being positive for up to a week after a bleed.

CT angiography will identify >95% of vascular causes of SAH.

You should be comfortable identifying different types of intracranial haemorrhage on different imaging modalities.

3. Describe the principles of medical and surgical management of this condition

Initial principles must include ABC and taking a thorough history, performing a full examination, and then arranging investigations to confirm the diagnosis.

Once confirmed, medical management includes flat bed rest and **HHH therapy** (see box). This essentially involves 3 L of intravenous fluids over 24 hours. In cases of aneurysmal SAH a **calcium channel antagonist** is used (commonly nimodipine given at 60 mg every 4 hours) and continued for 21 days. Anticonvulsants (e.g. phenytoin) should be considered.

Patients must then have regular neurological observations, preferably in a specialist neurosurgical centre. Aneurysms can be coiled or clipped (evidence from large trials such as ISAT and ISAT-II favour coiling). Further surgery is reserved for complications (see next section).

HHH therapy

⤢ Hypertension

⤢ Hypervolaemia

⤢ Haemodilution

3. Whilst on the ward the patient begins to slur her words and develops a right-sided weakness. Discuss possible complications of this condition and how they could be treated

This patient has likely developed **vasospasm**. Patients must be regularly assessed and altered neurology must be followed by a prompt CT scan. Vasospasm is managed via HHH therapy, with particular emphasis on hypertension. This may require a vasopressor such as metaraminol peripherally or noradrenaline centrally, often inducing systolic BP > 180 until symptoms resolve.

Rebleeding is managed as initial haemorrhages but can often be fatal.

Hydrocephalus is caused by RBC interfering with normal CSF circulation. If confirmed it must be treated via insertion of an external ventricular drain (EVD) to decompress the ventricular system. This can be removed as the patient recovers; however, many patients remain EVD dependant and should be considered for permanent CSF shunting (but not in the acute phase, as RBC will block the shunt catheter).

Other complications are prevented via judicious nursing/allied health professional involvement and regular haematological testing.

> **Complications of subarachnoid haemorrhage**
> * Rebleeding
> * Vasospasm
> * Hydrocephalus
> * Electrolyte abnormality
> * Systemic complications

4. How is the condition classified?

The most commonly used classifications in the UK are the **World Federation of Neurological Surgeons** (WFNS) (Table 53.1) and the **Fisher grading** (Table 53.2). The difference is that WFNS is based on GCS, whereas Fisher is based on CT appearances. This can be useful when discussing the case with a senior on the telephone as it can imply prognosis to an experienced neurosurgeon.

Table 53.1 WFNS grading of subarachnoid haemorrhage

Grade	GCS	Focal neurological deficit
1	15	Absent
2	13–14	Absent
3	13–14	Present
4	7–12	Present or absent
5	<7	Present or absent

Table 53.2 Fisher grading of subarachnoid haemorrhage

Grade	Appearance of haemorrhage
1	None evident
2	<1 mm thick
3	>1 mm thick
4	Any thickness with intraventricular haemorrhage or parenchymal extension

53.3 Cord compression

History
* Pain
* Paraesthesiae

↗ Weakness

↗ Bladder and bowel symptoms

↗ History of trauma

↗ Associated systemic illness

↗ Smoking

Examination

Inspect	• Vital signs
	• GCS
Move	• Tone
	• Power
Test	• Reflexes
	• Coordination
	• Sensation
	• Straight-leg raise
	• Proprioception
	• Vibration sense
	• Temperature sense
	• Clonus

Present

'A 51-year old man presents with acute leg numbness and inability to mobilize. He reports some difficulty initiating micturition and he has had periodic faecal incontinence. On questioning he reveals some weight loss over the last 2 months along with gradually worsening back pain. He has smoked 20 cigarettes a day for the last 30 years. On examination his GCS is 15 and he exhibits increased tone, brisk reflexes, and sustained ankle clonus in both lower limbs. He also has diffuse altered sensation in the lower limbs, with altered proprioception.'

Likely questions

1. Give a brief overview of the location and function of the main spinal cord pathways

The main cord pathways are the corticospinal tract, spinothalamic tract, and dorsal columns.

↗ The **corticospinal tract** arises from the primary motor cortex. Within the medulla, the majority of fibres cross to the contralateral side of the brainstem and spinal cord (known as the **pyramidal decussation**). These form the lateral corticospinal tracts. The remaining neurons cross the cord at the level of exit, and these travel in the anterior corticospinal tract.

↗ The **spinothalamic tract** is a purely sensory pathway, which carries modalities of pain, touch, temperature, and itch. The tract crosses the cord one or two levels above the point of entry, i.e. the neurons enter the cord on the ipsilateral side and ascend one or two levels via Lissauer's tract before synapsing and crossing to the contralateral side. The tract carries information to the thalamus.

↗ The **dorsal columns** are involved with transmission of fine touch, vibration, and proprioceptive information. This information travels within the fasciculus cuneatus and fasciculus gracilis before decussating in the medulla at the sensory decussation, forming the medial lemniscus.

Remember: spinal cord syndromes:

↗ Anterior cord syndrome

↗ Central cord syndrome

↗ Brown–Séquard

2. You suspect this patient has spinal cord compression. What investigations would you consider?

CT scanning will show bony changes around the spine. The most important investigation is **MRI scan** of the whole spine which will demonstrate signal change within the spinal cord. In this case, the patient may have malignant cord compression, therefore a **chest radiograph** and **CT chest, abdomen, and pelvis** for staging should be considered. Full blood tests, including **tumour markers** and a **myeloma screen** should be performed if indicated.

3. You are asked to consent the patient for a decompressive laminectomy. Describe the risks of surgery that you will discuss with the patient and his family

The purpose of the operation is to create room for the spinal cord by relieving pressure. The procedure involves a general anaesthetic. The operation involves stripping of the muscles and removal of the spinous process and lamina of the appropriate vertebra, along with the ligamentous structures. There is a small risk of damage to the nerve roots, which can result in new numbness or weakness. The dura can be damaged, resulting in CSF leak. There is a risk of wound infection. Nerves supplying the bladder and controlling sexual function can be damaged, resulting in incontinence or erectile dysfunction. A blood transfusion may be required. After the operation a drain may be in place for a short time.

4. In general terms, provide examples of pathologies that could present with spinal cord compression

Broadly speaking, they can be divided into congenital or acquired. Neoplastic causes can be primary or secondary. An infective cause may be represented by an abscess. Trauma could cause fractures or bleeding which could disrupt normal architecture and impinge on the cord. Extradural haemorrhage or infarction and subsequent swelling are examples of vascular causes. Ruptured intervertebral discs/osteophytes cover degenerative changes. Chronic inflammatory changes such as a granuloma are pertinent also.

Causes of cord compression
- ↗ Congenital
- ↗ Acquired:
  - Neoplastic
  - Metabolic
  - Infective
  - Traumatic
  - Autoimmune
  - Vascular
  - Inflammatory
  - Degenerative
  - Idiopathic

53.4 Traumatic head injury

History
- ↗ Mechanism of trauma
- ↗ Any safety equipment used (e.g. seatbelts/helmets)
- ↗ Unconsciousness
- ↗ Seizures
- ↗ Neurological deficit

Examination

Inspect   Primary and secondary survey

Test   • GCS
   • Baseline full neurological examination

Present

'This 27-year old man reports a gunshot wound to the head 6 years ago. He had no recollection of the incident and was told later he was intubated at the scene. There is a small frontal scar with a larger healed wound above the right ear. The patient is orientated but only scores 8 out of 10 on the Mini-Mental State Examination. There are no focal neurological defects.'

Likely questions

1. Describe your initial approach to the patient if you had been in the Emergency Department on the night of his injury

Initial approach should be around ATLS protocols, with a strict ABC primary survey, followed by secondary survey and adjunct to it

> All trauma scenarios in the examination should involve an early reference to ATLS™.

2. Following resuscitation, the patient was taken to theatre by the neurosurgeons. What are the general principles of any surgery to be performed?

The patient clearly had a severe brain injury. There is likely to be foreign material, including bone and dirt within the wound. Because of this there has to be a thorough debridement and exploration of the wound and the tract, removing any devitalized tissue and bone, with washout. The brain can be expected to swell, therefore it is important to consider decompression, in the form of a **craniectomy** with or without a **lobectomy**.

3. 1 day postoperatively, you are called to intensive care where the patient remains intubated and ventilated. The nursing staff inform you that his ICP has been 28 for the last 30 minutes. Outline your management options for raised ICP

It is important first to assess the patient for reversible causes of increased ICP. In the intubated and ventilated patient, adequacy of sedation must be assessed, as it may be inadequate. Is the patient having subclinical seizures requiring treatment? Is the patient pyrexial? Does he have any infection requiring treatment? This involves blood tests, which can also examine metabolic causes. Arterial blood gas sampling is important as it will show if the patient is hypoxic or hypercapnic—reversible causes. These can be treated by discussing ventilatory goals with the intensivist, who can alter the ventilator settings. Further medical treatment includes induced coma via thiopentone or phenobarbital. In the meantime the patient must have a head scan to exclude surgical causes, and it is useful at this point to consider an osmotic diuretic such as mannitol, which provides a temporary reduction in ICP while the cause is investigated. If a surgical cause such as hydrocephalus, cerebral oedema, or haematoma is revealed, surgical steps such as external ventricular drainage, decompressive craniectomy, or evacuation of clot can be considered. Principles are in place to maintain cerebral perfusion pressure (CPP).

CPP = MAP (mean arterial pressure) − ICP.

53.5 Multiple sclerosis

History

⤢ Paraesthesiae

⤢ Weakness

⤢ Spasms

↗ Ataxia

↗ Dysarthria

↗ Dysphagia

↗ Visual problems

↗ Fatigue

Examination

Move • Tone
 • Power

Test • Cranial nerves
 • Reflexes
 • Coordination
 • Sensation

Present

'This 28-year old woman reports a sudden onset of right leg weakness while playing netball. She has no significant medical history but recalls that following a party last year her left hand was numb for a few days and she had some double vision. Tone and reflexes are exaggerated on the right lower limb. The same limb is found to be weak. Plantar response is upgoing. Sensation is normal.'

Remember: multiple sclerosis can present with many different neurological signs.

Likely questions

1. What are the differential diagnoses?

Multiple sclerosis (MS) is the most likely diagnosis.

MS has a plethora of differential diagnoses. Remember the surgical sieve. Some examples include: inflammatory (systemic lupus erythematosus, vasculitis, sarcoidosis); infectious (Lyme disease, herpes zoster); genetic (mitochondrial disorders, CADASIL); metabolic (vitamin B_{12} deficiency), neoplastic (intracerebral primary and secondary tumours) and spinal (degenerative and vascular malformations).

2. What imaging would you request on this patient and what would you expect to see?

I would request an MRI scan of the brain and spine with gadolinium. In MS this would show **white matter changes** consistent with demyelination (called plaques). Gadolinium has the advantage of highlighting active lesions, which will be enhanced.

3. What further investigations are important to formulate a diagnosis?

Different criteria are required to diagnose MS, with the **McDonald** being the most widely used in the UK. This essentially requires clinical, radiological, and laboratory data highlighting lesions separate in time and space. On the face of history and MRI evidence, one would proceed to lumbar puncture (LP), specifically looking for **oligoclonal bands of IgG** in the CSF. Further tests include visual and sensory evoked potentials, in cases of optic nerve plaques.

53.6 Intracerebral tumour

History

↗ Weakness

↗ Confusion

↗ Seizure

↗ Paraesthesia

↗ Altered behaviour

↗ Headache

↗ Visual disturbance

Examination

Inspect Fundoscopy

Move • Tone
  • Power

Test • GCS
  • Reflexes

Present

'This 62-year old woman presents with collapse, tongue biting, and incontinence of urine. She was unresponsive for 2–3 minutes, with no abnormal movements. She has a history of depression but is otherwise well. She currently is confused, with no focal neurology although there is bilateral papilloedema.'

Likely questions

1. What is your initial management?

Initial management is an ABC approach, followed by blood tests including clotting screen and a group and save. Because there is evidence of seizures, an anticonvulsant such as phenytoin should be commenced. At this stage, one would consider imaging, with CT head being first line. In this case GCS is E4 V4 M6, but if the GCS was 8 or less an anaesthetist should be contacted as the patient ought to not be transferred anywhere without securing the airway.

2. Describe features of raised intracranial pressure

Raised ICP is characterized by headache that is worse in the morning, nausea and vomiting, altered conscious level, papilloedema, and visual disturbance.

3. A CT scan shows a space occupying lesion in the right temporal lobe with surrounding oedema. What drugs are useful to add at this point?

Steroids are useful in the treatment of oedema. Normally dexamethasone is given at a dose of 4 mg four times per day.

> **Always remember gastric protection when using steroids**

4. What treatment options are available?

The patient should be discussed with the on-call neurosurgical team. They may recommend that the patient be discussed at a multidisciplinary team meeting before formulating a management plan. Otherwise, treatment is essentially operative or nonoperative. Nonoperative management will include seizure control and management of cerebral oedema. There may be a case for radiological surveillance of lesions that are deemed to have a low grade. In suspected malignant lesions, a **staging CT scan** and tumour markers are useful adjuncts to treatment.

Operative management ranges from biopsy to complete excision; however, many lesions are unsuitable for complete excision because of their eloquent location within the brain or their diffuse nature. In this case debulking may be performed for symptom control.

This can be followed be radiotherapy or chemotherapy, which ought to be managed by a specialist neuro-oncology team if available. Patients must have sufficient information to decide about the management of their condition, as life expectancies can be short in high-grade tumours.

5. Discuss the aetiology of intracranial mass lesions?

The surgical sieve ought to be employed again. Congenital lesions ay be cystic in origin, acquired lesions include primary and secondary / benign and malignant neoplasms; Infective causes include intracranial abscess; Vascular causes include intracerebral haematomas and infarction; Inflammatory causes such as oedema; Traumatic brain contusions.

53.7 Extradural haematoma

History
- ➹ Mode of injury
- ➹ Seizures
- ➹ Headache
- ➹ Conscious level
- ➹ Alcohol consumption
- ➹ Weakness

Examination

Move Tone
Power

Test Reflexes
Cranial nerves

Present

'This 35-year old alcoholic man was admitted after drinking all day. He reportedly fell down a flight of stairs; he did not lose consciousness but has become increasingly drowsy and disorientated since. He takes medication for a longstanding depressive illness. On arrival his GCS was E3 V1 M5, but dropped to E1 V1 M1. His left pupil was fixed and dilated and he had blood coming from his left ear.'

Likely questions

1. What do you expect to see on a CT scan?

Extradural haematoma is classically a lens-shaped haematoma.

2. You correctly diagnose an extradural haemorrhage. What are your management steps?

In this case the patient requires urgent decompression of the haematoma in theatre. However, before that the patient requires intubation because his GCS is less than eight. Furthermore he requires blood tests including clotting profile and group and save, although failure to procure these ought not to delay the procedure. The patient is also at risk of seizures and ought to be commenced on an antiseizure medication such as phenytoin.

> Not all extradural haemorrhages require decompression, but this decision needs to be made by experienced neurosurgeons.

2. What are the longer-term management considerations in this patient?

In the initial postoperative period the patient is at risk of withdrawal from alcohol, therefore should be commenced on intravenous B vitamins, followed by oral equivalents. Additionally, he ought to have benzodiazepines such as chlordiazepoxide for withdrawal reactions. The patient will require inpatient rehabilitation from allied health professionals and will likely require referral to a neurorehabilitation centre for longer-term management. Furthermore, he would benefit from alcohol cessation counselling.

> **Always think about nonsurgical issues when asked this kind of question.**

3. Why is the bloody discharge from the ear concerning? What else could a patient exhibit and how can it be managed?

This is concerning as it may represent a basal skull fracture. Other signs include Battle's sign and racoon (or panda) eyes. In addition to blood from the ear, CSF may also leak from the ear or nose in the form of CSF oto/rhinorrhoea. Patients may complain of a salty taste in the throat. Specimens ought to be collected from any fluid leaking and sent for analysis. CSF will be positive for tau protein. Patients should have a fine-cut CT scan of the skull base and this could be discussed with the maxillofacial team to decide if further input is needed. CSF leaks often resolve spontaneously within 2 weeks; however, if not, they may require repair by the neurosurgery or ENT unit. Some units also consider antibiotics for CSF leak.

53.8 Spinal cord injury

History

⬈ Mechanism of injury

⬈ Situation

⬈ Did the patient walk at the scene?

⬈ Has there been a change in neurology?

⬈ Were spinal precautions maintained?

⬈ Weakness

⬈ Paraesthesia

⬈ Altered conscious level

Examination

Move   Tone
           Power

Test   Reflexes
           Coordination
           Sensation

Present

'This 22-year old woman was admitted after diving into a shallow pool. She has been drinking heavily. On examination she has blood pressure of 94/68 which does not respond to fluids, with a pulse of 75. She has flaccid paralysis of the lower limbs, reflexes are absent. She has absent sensation below the nipple line. There are no other obvious injuries.'

Likely questions

1. What are your initial management priorities?

The patient must be assessed from an ATLS point of view, with particular emphasis on cervical spine control in this instance. The patient requires investigations, namely CT scan of the head and spine and MRI scan of the spine at least.

2. What is the likely level of injury and how do you reach this conclusion?

The level is likely T4, as signified by the sensory level at the nipple line.

3. Why does her hypotension not respond to fluids?

The patient likely has neurogenic shock. It results from loss of autonomic and motor reflexes below the level of injury. Vessel walls relax without autonomic stimulation, resulting in a sudden decrease in peripheral vascular resistance, leading to vasodilation and hypotension.

4. What are the medium to long-term management strategies for these patients?

Despite the spinal cord injury, consideration should be given to stabilizing any fractures present to facilitate early rehabilitation and prevention of systemic complications from bed rest and immobilization. Furthermore, this patient is at risk of autonomic dysreflexia, which is characterized by unchecked sympathetic stimulation below the level of injury due to a loss of cranial regulation. This can lead to extreme hypertension, loss of bladder/bowel control, sweating, and headaches. The patient will require referral and transfer to a specialist spinal cord injury centre, which is best placed to manage these complications.

Chapter 54 **Common neurosurgical tests and signs**

The neurological clinical examination stations can seem particularly daunting, but having a clear structure can help. Examiners often speak of looking for a candidate to be 'slick' ... so practise!

Often neurological **illness** can produce an altered conscious level without producing a focal neurological **deficit**. However, **structural** neural damage (e.g. infarction, haematoma, tumours) can often result in profound changes. The ability to detect these and more subtle changes can distinguish between an average and an excellent candidate. This chapter assumes the candidate can perform a basic neurological examination but will highlight some extra tests that may enhance a candidate's performance when applied appropriately.

54.1 Before you start

Look at the patient:

↗ Abnormal gait

↗ Altered speech

↗ Involuntary movements

↗ Posture

Gait abnormalities

↗ Festinating

↗ Antalgic

↗ Ataxic

↗ Hemiparetic

↗ Footdrop

↗ Apraxic

54.2 Head and neck tests and signs

Dysarthria

↗ Poor articulation due to impaired motor control of components of speech

Dysphasia

↗ Language disorder, not related to the physical component of speech

Lhermitte's sign

↗ Passive flexion of the neck produces shooting pain into the limbs, which the patient often describes as being like an 'electric shock'

Kernig's sign

↗ Test for neck stiffness—can you passively flex the patient's neck from the bed to touch their chest?

Kernig's test

A further test of meningeal irritation.

↗ Lie the patient flat and flex one of the patient's legs at the knee and hip

↗ Try to straighten the leg

↗ If the contralateral hip flexes, the test is positive

Optic nerve

Remember that examination of the optic nerve involves more than fundoscopy and visual fields

---

CN III examination

↗ Fundoscopy

↗ Visual fields

> ↗ Pupillary response
> ↗ Colour vision
> ↗ Accommodation
> ↗ Visual acuity

Trigeminal nerve

↗ When testing the trigeminal nerve, remember the corneal reflex and the jaw jerk

Schirmer's test

↗ Unlikely that this will be asked, as it takes 5 minutes to perform, with the special paper under the lower eyelid

> Schirmer's tests are favoured in medical school OSCE examinations and candidates have been known to be asked about them in the iMRCS.

Rinne's test

↗ Compares bone conduction with air conduction

↗ Use a vibrating tuning fork with a frequency of 512 Hz on the mastoid process, then hold it next to the external auditory meatus—air conduction should be louder

Weber's test

↗ Place the vibrating tuning fork on the centre of the forehead. The perception of sound should remain on the midline

The Weber test is best thought of as a supplementary test as it can detect either a unilateral conductive or a sensorineural hearing loss.

> In neurosurgery, unilateral senorineural hearing loss is **acoustic neuroma** until proven otherwise.

Hallpike's test

This test for positional nystagmus is rarely used in reality.

↗ With the patient lying supine on an examination couch, the head is supported lying over the end of the couch

↗ Lower the head below horizontal and turn to either side to induce nystagmus

Oculocephalic reflex

This test of vestibular function is also known as the doll's eye reflex, which neatly describes the appearance.

↗ With the patient supine, rotate the head back and forth

↗ The eyes should remain looking ahead

Oculovestibular reflex

A further test of vestibular function, again rarely used in noncomatose patients.

↗ The external auditory canal is irrigated with water at 30 °C, inducing nystagmus in an intact brainstem

54.3 Peripheral tests

Hoffman's sign

An upper motor neuron sign.

↗ Allow the patient's hand to rest on yours by the distal interphalangeal joint of the middle finger

⚡ Flick the distal phalynx sharply downwards and observe for the thumb jerking

Other reflexes to consider if you believe a patient to be hyper-reflexic are finger jerks, pectoral jerks, and deltoid jerks.

Joint position sense

This is included here as it is often performed incorrectly.

The important thing to remember is to hold the joint being tested at the side, otherwise the patient will feel the upward or downward pressure and may be able to cheat your examination results. The dorsal columns must be intact for joint position to be maintained.

Vibration sense

A further test of dorsal columns.

⚡ Remember to use the 128-Hz tuning fork as opposed to the one used for Rinne's and Weber's tests

⚡ Use bony prominences such as the medial or lateral malleoli of the ankle joint

Grasp reflex

⚡ Run fingers across the palm of the patient, inducing a grasping motion

This reflex, which is traditionally associated with neonates, can return in elderly patients with cerebral atrophy or functional illness.

54.4 Sensory cortex tests

These tests assess the sensory cortex alone, and cannot be performed if any of the peripheral sensory pathways (e.g. spinothalamic tract) are impaired. It is therefore a useful functional assessment in a patient with an intracerebral tumour indicating how the lesion affects everyday function.

Stereognosis

⚡ Place objects into the patient's hands (with eyes closed) and ask the patient to identify each object

⚡ Failure to complete this demonstrates **astereognosis**

Graphaesthesia

⚡ Again with the eyes closed, trace a letter or number onto the patient's hand and have them repeat it to you

Point localization

⚡ With eyes closed, can patients identify which part of the body is being touched?

Apraxia

⚡ Can be constructional, where patients are asked to copy a shape (as in the Mini-Mental Test score), or dressing, which is self-explanatory (i.e. patients will struggle with buttons, etc.)

Dyscalculia

⚡ Again represented in the Mini-Mental Test: can patients perform subtraction (e.g. serial sevens)?

Sensory inattention

⚡ Have the patient close their eyes and touch left or right hand and ask the patient to identify which hand is touched

Chapter 55 **Brainstem death**

This is a common topic in the exam and one that lends itself to the scenario set-up of the iMRCS OSCE.

55.1 Definition

This is a situation in which there is an irreversible failure of brainstem function.

The rules governing under what circumstances a patient can be tested and by whom and how were laid out in a 1976 consensus publication following a conference of the Royal Colleges.

55.2 Patient conditions

↗ No depressant drugs

- ◆ In practice, for patients on the intensive care unit, this means that adequate time must elapse without any sedative agents

↗ Core body temperature must not be less than 35 °C

↗ No neuromuscular blockade

↗ Metabolic or endocrine causes must be excluded

↗ Cause of patient's condition must be known and compatible with irreversible brain damage

55.3 Doctor criteria

↗ These tests must be carried out by two GMC-registered doctors with expertise in the field of brain injury

↗ One doctor must be a consultant, the other a senior trainee or consultant

↗ Doctors may perform tests together or separately

↗ Adequate time must have elapsed from onset of the condition to ensure the preconditions are met without doubt

55.4 Brainstem death criteria

Pupillary reflex

↗ No pupillary response to light

↗ Negative corneal reflex (no movement of eyelid on stimulation of cornea)

Motor reflexes

↗ No movement in muscles supplied by cranial nerves in response to a central painful stimulus (e.g. supraorbital painful stimulus)

Vestibulo-ocular reflex

↗ Caloric testing—no eye movement on injection of 50 mL of ice-cold water into the external acoustic meatus (when brainstem function is preserved, eyes will deviate towards the tested ear)

Gag reflex

↗ No response to bronchial stimulation (here you are looking for any cough response)

Respiratory movements

↗ No respiratory effort after disconnection from endotracheal tube (oxygenation usually maintained with 6 L O_2 and Pco_2 kept above 6.65 kPa)

Certification of death is made once brainstem death is established, with the time of death being the time that the second tests were completed.

Index